Mometrix
TEST PREPARATION

Certified Disability Management Specialist Exam

Secrets Study Guide

I0889382

DEAR FUTURE EXAM SUCCESS STORY

First of all, **THANK YOU** for purchasing Mometrix study materials!

Second, congratulations! You are one of the few determined test-takers who are committed to doing whatever it takes to excel on your exam. **You have come to the right place.** We developed these study materials with one goal in mind: to deliver you the information you need in a format that's concise and easy to use.

In addition to optimizing your guide for the content of the test, we've outlined our recommended steps for breaking down the preparation process into small, attainable goals so you can make sure you stay on track.

We've also analyzed the entire test-taking process, identifying the most common pitfalls and showing how you can overcome them and be ready for any curveball the test throws you.

Standardized testing is one of the biggest obstacles on your road to success, which only increases the importance of doing well in the high-pressure, high-stakes environment of test day. Your results on this test could have a significant impact on your future, and this guide provides the information and practical advice to help you achieve your full potential on test day.

Your success is our success

We would love to hear from you! If you would like to share the story of your exam success or if you have any questions or comments in regard to our products, please contact us at **800-673-8175** or **support@mometrix.com**.

Thanks again for your business and we wish you continued success!

Sincerely,
The Mometrix Test Preparation Team

Written and edited by the Mometrix Exam Secrets Test Prep Team
Printed in the United States of America

TABLE OF CONTENTS

Introduction

Thank you for purchasing this resource! You have made the choice to prepare yourself for a test that could have a huge impact on your future, and this guide is designed to help you be fully ready for test day. Obviously, it's important to have a solid understanding of the test material, but you also need to be prepared for the unique environment and stressors of the test, so that you can perform to the best of your abilities.

For this purpose, the first section that appears in this guide is the **Secret Keys**. We've devoted countless hours to meticulously researching what works and what doesn't, and we've boiled down our findings to the five most impactful steps you can take to improve your performance on the test. We start at the beginning with study planning and move through the preparation process, all the way to the testing strategies that will help you get the most out of what you know when you're finally sitting in front of the test.

We recommend that you start preparing for your test as far in advance as possible. However, if you've bought this guide as a last-minute study resource and only have a few days before your test, we recommend that you skip over the first two Secret Keys since they address a long-term study plan.

If you struggle with **test anxiety**, we strongly encourage you to check out our recommendations for how you can overcome it. Test anxiety is a formidable foe, but it can be beaten, and we want to make sure you have the tools you need to defeat it.

Secret Key 1: Plan Big, Study Small

There's a lot riding on your performance. If you want to ace this test, you're going to need to keep your skills sharp and the material fresh in your mind. You need a plan that lets you review everything you need to know while still fitting in your schedule. We'll break this strategy down into three categories.

Information Organization

Start with the information you already have: the official test outline. From this, you can make a complete list of all the concepts you need to cover before the test. Organize these concepts into groups that can be studied together, and create a list of any related vocabulary you need to learn so you can brush up on any difficult terms. You'll want to keep this vocabulary list handy once you actually start studying since you may need to add to it along the way.

Time Management

Once you have your set of study concepts, decide how to spread them out over the time you have left before the test. Break your study plan into small, clear goals so you have a manageable task for each day and know exactly what you're doing. Then just focus on one small step at a time. When you manage your time this way, you don't need to spend hours at a time studying. Studying a small block of content for a short period each day helps you retain information better and avoid stressing over how much you have left to do. You can relax knowing that you have a plan to cover everything in time. In order for this strategy to be effective though, you have to start studying early and stick to your schedule. Avoid the exhaustion and futility that comes from last-minute cramming!

Study Environment

The environment you study in has a big impact on your learning. Studying in a coffee shop, while probably more enjoyable, is not likely to be as fruitful as studying in a quiet room. It's important to keep distractions to a minimum. You're only planning to study for a short block of time, so make the most of it. Don't pause to check your phone or get up to find a snack. It's also important to **avoid multitasking**. Research has consistently shown that multitasking will make your studying dramatically less effective. Your study area should also be comfortable and well-lit so you don't have the distraction of straining your eyes or sitting on an uncomfortable chair.

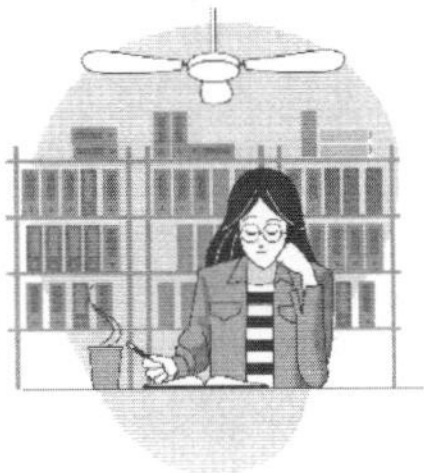

The time of day you study is also important. You want to be rested and alert. Don't wait until just before bedtime. Study when you'll be most likely to comprehend and remember. Even better, if you know what time of day your test will be, set that time aside for study. That way your brain will be used to working on that subject at that specific time and you'll have a better chance of recalling information.

Finally, it can be helpful to team up with others who are studying for the same test. Your actual studying should be done in as isolated an environment as possible, but the work of organizing the information and setting up the study plan can be divided up. In between study sessions, you can discuss with your teammates the concepts that you're all studying and quiz each other on the details. Just be sure that your teammates are as serious about the test as you are. If you find that your study time is being replaced with social time, you might need to find a new team.

Secret Key 2: Make Your Studying Count

You're devoting a lot of time and effort to preparing for this test, so you want to be absolutely certain it will pay off. This means doing more than just reading the content and hoping you can remember it on test day. It's important to make every minute of study count. There are two main areas you can focus on to make your studying count.

Retention

It doesn't matter how much time you study if you can't remember the material. You need to make sure you are retaining the concepts. To check your retention of the information you're learning, try recalling it at later times with minimal prompting. Try carrying around flashcards and glance at one or two from time to time or ask a friend who's also studying for the test to quiz you.

To enhance your retention, look for ways to put the information into practice so that you can apply it rather than simply recalling it. If you're using the information in practical ways, it will be much easier to remember. Similarly, it helps to solidify a concept in your mind if you're not only reading it to yourself but also explaining it to someone else. Ask a friend to let you teach them about a concept you're a little shaky on (or speak aloud to an imaginary audience if necessary). As you try to summarize, define, give examples, and answer your friend's questions, you'll understand the concepts better and they will stay with you longer. Finally, step back for a big picture view and ask yourself how each piece of information fits with the whole subject. When you link the different concepts together and see them working together as a whole, it's easier to remember the individual components.

Finally, practice showing your work on any multi-step problems, even if you're just studying. Writing out each step you take to solve a problem will help solidify the process in your mind, and you'll be more likely to remember it during the test.

Modality

Modality simply refers to the means or method by which you study. Choosing a study modality that fits your own individual learning style is crucial. No two people learn best in exactly the same way, so it's important to know your strengths and use them to your advantage.

For example, if you learn best by visualization, focus on visualizing a concept in your mind and draw an image or a diagram. Try color-coding your notes, illustrating them, or creating symbols that will trigger your mind to recall a learned concept. If you learn best by hearing or discussing information, find a study partner who learns the same way or read aloud to yourself. Think about how to put the information in your own words. Imagine that you are giving a lecture on the topic and record yourself so you can listen to it later.

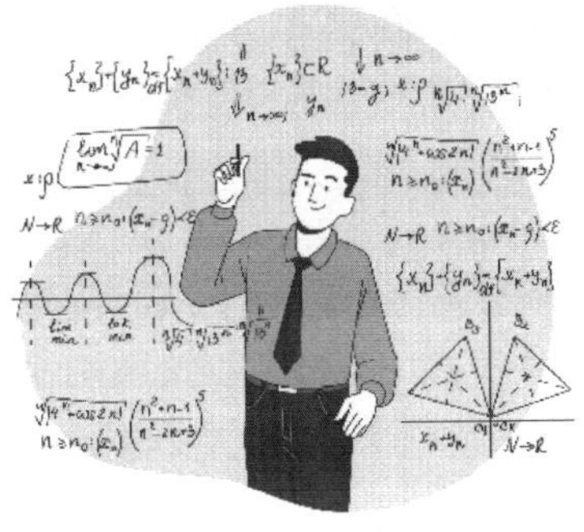

For any learning style, flashcards can be helpful. Organize the information so you can take advantage of spare moments to review. Underline key words or phrases. Use different colors for different categories. Mnemonic devices (such as creating a short list in which every item starts with the same letter) can also help with retention. Find what works best for you and use it to store the information in your mind most effectively and easily.

Secret Key 3: Practice the Right Way

Your success on test day depends not only on how many hours you put into preparing, but also on whether you prepared the right way. It's good to check along the way to see if your studying is paying off. One of the most effective ways to do this is by taking practice tests to evaluate your progress. Practice tests are useful because they show exactly where you need to improve. Every time you take a practice test, pay special attention to these three groups of questions:

- The questions you got wrong
- The questions you had to guess on, even if you guessed right
- The questions you found difficult or slow to work through

This will show you exactly what your weak areas are, and where you need to devote more study time. Ask yourself why each of these questions gave you trouble. Was it because you didn't understand the material? Was it because you didn't remember the vocabulary? Do you need more repetitions on this type of question to build speed and confidence? Dig into those questions and figure out how you can strengthen your weak areas as you go back to review the material.

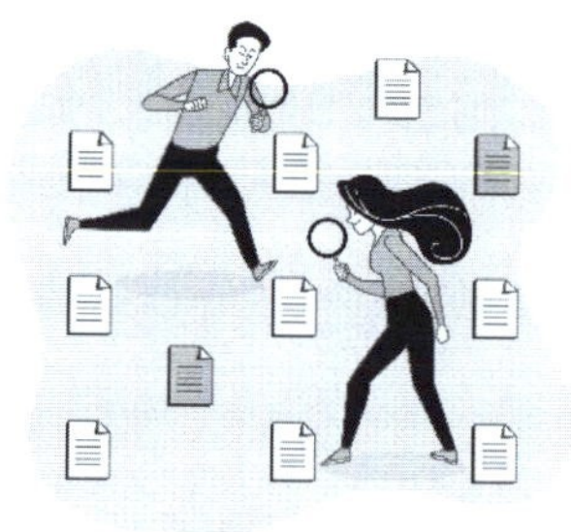

Additionally, many practice tests have a section explaining the answer choices. It can be tempting to read the explanation and think that you now have a good understanding of the concept. However, an explanation likely only covers part of the question's broader context. Even if the explanation makes perfect sense, **go back and investigate** every concept related to the question until you're positive you have a thorough understanding.

As you go along, keep in mind that the practice test is just that: practice. Memorizing these questions and answers will not be very helpful on the actual test because it is unlikely to have any of the same exact questions. If you only know the right answers to the sample questions, you won't be prepared for the real thing. **Study the concepts** until you understand them fully, and then you'll be able to answer any question that shows up on the test.

It's important to wait on the practice tests until you're ready. If you take a test on your first day of study, you may be overwhelmed by the amount of material covered and how much you need to learn. Work up to it gradually.

On test day, you'll need to be prepared for answering questions, managing your time, and using the test-taking strategies you've learned. It's a lot to balance, like a mental marathon that will have a big impact on your future. Like training for a marathon, you'll need to start slowly and work your way up. When test day arrives, you'll be ready.

Start with the strategies you've read in the first two Secret Keys—plan your course and study in the way that works best for you. If you have time, consider using multiple study resources to get different approaches to the same concepts. It can be helpful to see difficult concepts from more than one angle. Then find a good source for practice tests. Many times, the test website will suggest potential study resources or provide sample tests.

Practice Test Strategy

If you're able to find at least three practice tests, we recommend this strategy:

Untimed and Open-Book Practice

Take the first test with no time constraints and with your notes and study guide handy. Take your time and focus on applying the strategies you've learned.

Timed and Open-Book Practice

Take the second practice test open-book as well, but set a timer and practice pacing yourself to finish in time.

Timed and Closed-Book Practice

Take any other practice tests as if it were test day. Set a timer and put away your study materials. Sit at a table or desk in a quiet room, imagine yourself at the testing center, and answer questions as quickly and accurately as possible.

Keep repeating timed and closed-book tests on a regular basis until you run out of practice tests or it's time for the actual test. Your mind will be ready for the schedule and stress of test day, and you'll be able to focus on recalling the material you've learned.

Secret Key 4: Pace Yourself

Once you're fully prepared for the material on the test, your biggest challenge on test day will be managing your time. Just knowing that the clock is ticking can make you panic even if you have plenty of time left. Work on pacing yourself so you can build confidence against the time constraints of the exam. Pacing is a difficult skill to master, especially in a high-pressure environment, so **practice is vital**.

Set time expectations for your pace based on how much time is available. For example, if a section has 60 questions and the time limit is 30 minutes, you know you have to average 30 seconds or less per question in order to answer them all. Although 30 seconds is the hard limit, set 25 seconds per question as your goal, so you reserve extra time to spend on harder questions. When you budget extra time for the harder questions, you no longer have any reason to stress when those questions take longer to answer.

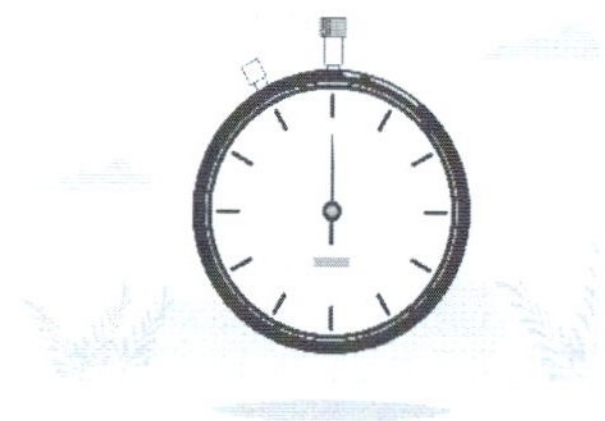

Don't let this time expectation distract you from working through the test at a calm, steady pace, but keep it in mind so you don't spend too much time on any one question. Recognize that taking extra time on one question you don't understand may keep you from answering two that you do understand later in the test. If your time limit for a question is up and you're still not sure of the answer, mark it and move on, and come back to it later if the time and the test format allow. If the testing format doesn't allow you to return to earlier questions, just make an educated guess; then put it out of your mind and move on.

On the easier questions, be careful not to rush. It may seem wise to hurry through them so you have more time for the challenging ones, but it's not worth missing one if you know the concept and just didn't take the time to read the question fully. Work efficiently but make sure you understand the question and have looked at all of the answer choices, since more than one may seem right at first.

Even if you're paying attention to the time, you may find yourself a little behind at some point. You should speed up to get back on track, but do so wisely. Don't panic; just take a few seconds less on each question until you're caught up. Don't guess without thinking, but do look through the answer choices and eliminate any you know are wrong. If you can get down to two choices, it is often worthwhile to guess from those. Once you've chosen an answer, move on and don't dwell on any that you skipped or had to hurry through. If a question was taking too long, chances are it was one of the harder ones, so you weren't as likely to get it right anyway.

On the other hand, if you find yourself getting ahead of schedule, it may be beneficial to slow down a little. The more quickly you work, the more likely you are to make a careless mistake that will affect your score. You've budgeted time for each question, so don't be afraid to spend that time. Practice an efficient but careful pace to get the most out of the time you have.

Secret Key 5: Have a Plan for Guessing

When you're taking the test, you may find yourself stuck on a question. Some of the answer choices seem better than others, but you don't see the one answer choice that is obviously correct. What do you do?

The scenario described above is very common, yet most test takers have not effectively prepared for it. Developing and practicing a plan for guessing may be one of the single most effective uses of your time as you get ready for the exam.

In developing your plan for guessing, there are three questions to address:

- When should you start the guessing process?
- How should you narrow down the choices?
- Which answer should you choose?

When to Start the Guessing Process

Unless your plan for guessing is to select C every time (which, despite its merits, is not what we recommend), you need to leave yourself enough time to apply your answer elimination strategies. Since you have a limited amount of time for each question, that means that if you're going to give yourself the best shot at guessing correctly, you have to decide quickly whether or not you will guess.

Of course, the best-case scenario is that you don't have to guess at all, so first, see if you can answer the question based on your knowledge of the subject and basic reasoning skills. Focus on the key words in the question and try to jog your memory of related topics. Give yourself a chance to bring the knowledge to mind, but once you realize that you don't have (or you can't access) the knowledge you need to answer the question, it's time to start the guessing process.

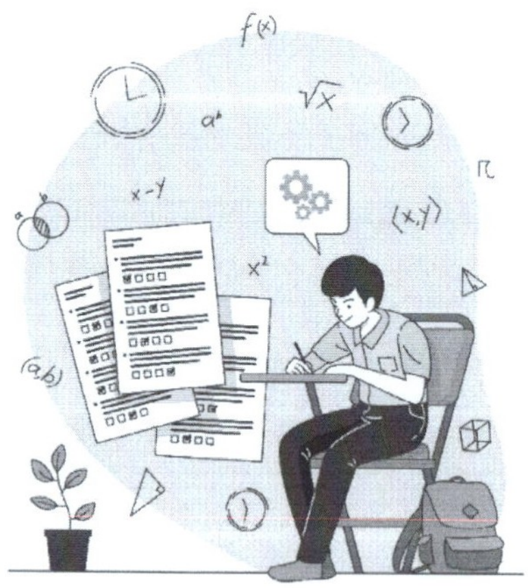

It's almost always better to start the guessing process too early than too late. It only takes a few seconds to remember something and answer the question from knowledge. Carefully eliminating wrong answer choices takes longer. Plus, going through the process of eliminating answer choices can actually help jog your memory.

Summary: Start the guessing process as soon as you decide that you can't answer the question based on your knowledge.

How to Narrow Down the Choices

The next chapter in this book (**Test-Taking Strategies**) includes a wide range of strategies for how to approach questions and how to look for answer choices to eliminate. You will definitely want to read those carefully, practice them, and figure out which ones work best for you. Here though, we're going to address a mindset rather than a particular strategy.

Your odds of guessing an answer correctly depend on how many options you are choosing from.

Number of options left	5	4	3	2	1
Odds of guessing correctly	20%	25%	33%	50%	100%

You can see from this chart just how valuable it is to be able to eliminate incorrect answers and make an educated guess, but there are two things that many test takers do that cause them to miss out on the benefits of guessing:

- Accidentally eliminating the correct answer
- Selecting an answer based on an impression

We'll look at the first one here, and the second one in the next section.

To avoid accidentally eliminating the correct answer, we recommend a thought exercise called **the $5 challenge**. In this challenge, you only eliminate an answer choice from contention if you are willing to bet $5 on it being wrong. Why $5? Five dollars is a small but not insignificant amount of money. It's an amount you could afford to lose but wouldn't want to throw away. And while losing $5 once might not hurt too much, doing it twenty times will set you back $100. In the same way, each small decision you make—eliminating a choice here, guessing on a question there—won't by itself impact your score very much, but when you put them all together, they can make a big difference. By holding each answer choice elimination decision to a higher standard, you can reduce the risk of accidentally eliminating the correct answer.

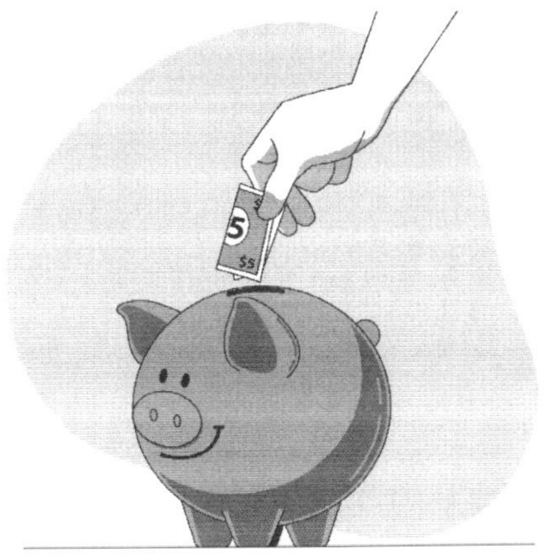

The $5 challenge can also be applied in a positive sense: If you are willing to bet $5 that an answer choice *is* correct, go ahead and mark it as correct.

Summary: Only eliminate an answer choice if you are willing to bet $5 that it is wrong.

Which Answer to Choose

You're taking the test. You've run into a hard question and decided you'll have to guess. You've eliminated all the answer choices you're willing to bet $5 on. Now you have to pick an answer. Why do we even need to talk about this? Why can't you just pick whichever one you feel like when the time comes?

The answer to these questions is that if you don't come into the test with a plan, you'll rely on your impression to select an answer choice, and if you do that, you risk falling into a trap. The test writers know that everyone who takes their test will be guessing on some of the questions, so they intentionally write wrong answer choices to seem plausible. You still have to pick an answer though, and if the wrong answer choices are designed to look right, how can you ever be sure that you're not falling for their trap? The best solution we've found to this dilemma is to take the decision out of your hands entirely. Here is the process we recommend:

Once you've eliminated any choices that you are confident (willing to bet $5) are wrong, select the first remaining choice as your answer.

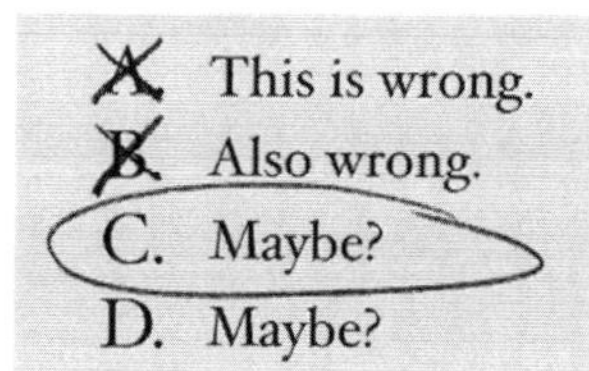

Whether you choose to select the first remaining choice, the second, or the last, the important thing is that you use some preselected standard. Using this approach guarantees that you will not be enticed into selecting an answer choice that looks right, because you are not basing your decision on how the answer choices look.

This is not meant to make you question your knowledge. Instead, it is to help you recognize the difference between your knowledge and your impressions. There's a huge difference between thinking an answer is right because of what you know, and thinking an answer is right because it looks or sounds like it should be right.

Summary: To ensure that your selection is appropriately random, make a predetermined selection from among all answer choices you have not eliminated.

Test-Taking Strategies

This section contains a list of test-taking strategies that you may find helpful as you work through the test. By taking what you know and applying logical thought, you can maximize your chances of answering any question correctly!

It is very important to realize that every question is different and every person is different: no single strategy will work on every question, and no single strategy will work for every person. That's why we've included all of them here, so you can try them out and determine which ones work best for different types of questions and which ones work best for you.

Question Strategies

☑ Read Carefully

Read the question and the answer choices carefully. Don't miss the question because you misread the terms. You have plenty of time to read each question thoroughly and make sure you understand what is being asked. Yet a happy medium must be attained, so don't waste too much time. You must read carefully and efficiently.

☑ Contextual Clues

Look for contextual clues. If the question includes a word you are not familiar with, look at the immediate context for some indication of what the word might mean. Contextual clues can often give you all the information you need to decipher the meaning of an unfamiliar word. Even if you can't determine the meaning, you may be able to narrow down the possibilities enough to make a solid guess at the answer to the question.

☑ Prefixes

If you're having trouble with a word in the question or answer choices, try dissecting it. Take advantage of every clue that the word might include. Prefixes can be a huge help. Usually, they allow you to determine a basic meaning. *Pre-* means before, *post-* means after, *pro-* is positive, *de-* is negative. From prefixes, you can get an idea of the general meaning of the word and try to put it into context.

☑ Hedge Words

Watch out for critical hedge words, such as *likely, may, can, often, almost, mostly, usually, generally, rarely,* and *sometimes*. Question writers insert these hedge phrases to cover every possibility. Often an answer choice will be wrong simply because it leaves no room for exception. Be on guard for answer choices that have definitive words such as *exactly* and *always*.

✅ Switchback Words

Stay alert for *switchbacks*. These are the words and phrases frequently used to alert you to shifts in thought. The most common switchback words are *but*, *although*, and *however*. Others include *nevertheless*, *on the other hand*, *even though*, *while*, *in spite of*, *despite*, and *regardless of*. Switchback words are important to catch because they can change the direction of the question or an answer choice.

✅ Face Value

When in doubt, use common sense. Accept the situation in the problem at face value. Don't read too much into it. These problems will not require you to make wild assumptions. If you have to go beyond creativity and warp time or space in order to have an answer choice fit the question, then you should move on and consider the other answer choices. These are normal problems rooted in reality. The applicable relationship or explanation may not be readily apparent, but it is there for you to figure out. Use your common sense to interpret anything that isn't clear.

Answer Choice Strategies

✅ Answer Selection

The most thorough way to pick an answer choice is to identify and eliminate wrong answers until only one is left, then confirm it is the correct answer. Sometimes an answer choice may immediately seem right, but be careful. The test writers will usually put more than one reasonable answer choice on each question, so take a second to read all of them and make sure that the other choices are not equally obvious. As long as you have time left, it is better to read every answer choice than to pick the first one that looks right without checking the others.

✅ Answer Choice Families

An answer choice family consists of two (in rare cases, three) answer choices that are very similar in construction and cannot all be true at the same time. If you see two answer choices that are direct opposites or parallels, one of them is usually the correct answer. For instance, if one answer choice says that quantity x increases and another either says that quantity x decreases (opposite) or says that quantity y increases (parallel), then those answer choices would fall into the same family. An answer choice that doesn't match the construction of the answer choice family is more likely to be incorrect. Most questions will not have answer choice families, but when they do appear, you should be prepared to recognize them.

✅ Eliminate Answers

Eliminate answer choices as soon as you realize they are wrong, but make sure you consider all possibilities. If you are eliminating answer choices and realize that the last one you are left with is also wrong, don't panic. Start over and consider each choice again. There may be something you missed the first time that you will realize on the second pass.

⊘ Avoid Fact Traps

Don't be distracted by an answer choice that is factually true but doesn't answer the question. You are looking for the choice that answers the question. Stay focused on what the question is asking for so you don't accidentally pick an answer that is true but incorrect. Always go back to the question and make sure the answer choice you've selected actually answers the question and is not merely a true statement.

⊘ Extreme Statements

In general, you should avoid answers that put forth extreme actions as standard practice or proclaim controversial ideas as established fact. An answer choice that states the "process should be used in certain situations, if…" is much more likely to be correct than one that states the "process should be discontinued completely." The first is a calm rational statement and doesn't even make a definitive, uncompromising stance, using a hedge word *if* to provide wiggle room, whereas the second choice is far more extreme.

⊘ Benchmark

As you read through the answer choices and you come across one that seems to answer the question well, mentally select that answer choice. This is not your final answer, but it's the one that will help you evaluate the other answer choices. The one that you selected is your benchmark or standard for judging each of the other answer choices. Every other answer choice must be compared to your benchmark. That choice is correct until proven otherwise by another answer choice beating it. If you find a better answer, then that one becomes your new benchmark. Once you've decided that no other choice answers the question as well as your benchmark, you have your final answer.

⊘ Predict the Answer

Before you even start looking at the answer choices, it is often best to try to predict the answer. When you come up with the answer on your own, it is easier to avoid distractions and traps because you will know exactly what to look for. The right answer choice is unlikely to be word-for-word what you came up with, but it should be a close match. Even if you are confident that you have the right answer, you should still take the time to read each option before moving on.

General Strategies

⊘ Tough Questions

If you are stumped on a problem or it appears too hard or too difficult, don't waste time. Move on! Remember though, if you can quickly check for obviously incorrect answer choices, your chances of guessing correctly are greatly improved. Before you completely give up, at least try to knock out a couple of possible answers. Eliminate what you can and then guess at the remaining answer choices before moving on.

⊘ Check Your Work

Since you will probably not know every term listed and the answer to every question, it is important that you get credit for the ones that you do know. Don't miss any questions through careless mistakes. If at all possible, try to take a second to look back over your answer selection and make sure you've selected the correct answer choice and haven't made a costly careless mistake (such as marking an answer choice that you didn't mean to mark). This quick double check should more than pay for itself in caught mistakes for the time it costs.

⊘ Pace Yourself

It's easy to be overwhelmed when you're looking at a page full of questions; your mind is confused and full of random thoughts, and the clock is ticking down faster than you would like. Calm down and maintain the pace that you have set for yourself. Especially as you get down to the last few minutes of the test, don't let the small numbers on the clock make you panic. As long as you are on track by monitoring your pace, you are guaranteed to have time for each question.

⊘ Don't Rush

It is very easy to make errors when you are in a hurry. Maintaining a fast pace in answering questions is pointless if it makes you miss questions that you would have gotten right otherwise. Test writers like to include distracting information and wrong answers that seem right. Taking a little extra time to avoid careless mistakes can make all the difference in your test score. Find a pace that allows you to be confident in the answers that you select.

⊘ Keep Moving

Panicking will not help you pass the test, so do your best to stay calm and keep moving. Taking deep breaths and going through the answer elimination steps you practiced can help to break through a stress barrier and keep your pace.

Final Notes

The combination of a solid foundation of content knowledge and the confidence that comes from practicing your plan for applying that knowledge is the key to maximizing your performance on test day. As your foundation of content knowledge is built up and strengthened, you'll find that the strategies included in this chapter become more and more effective in helping you quickly sift through the distractions and traps of the test to isolate the correct answer.

Now that you're preparing to move forward into the test content chapters of this book, be sure to keep your goal in mind. As you read, think about how you will be able to apply this information on the test. If you've already seen sample questions for the test and you have an idea of the question format and style, try to come up with questions of your own that you can answer based on what you're reading. This will give you valuable practice applying your knowledge in the same ways you can expect to on test day.

Good luck and good studying!

Disability and Work Interruption Case Management

Disability and Impairment

A disability refers to an inability to perform daily activities due to an accident or illness. These activities can be either job related or part of the daily activities of living such as bathing, feeding, dressing, walking, or running. Impairment refers to the abnormal loss of a function whether it is physical or mental. A disability can be a disease, illness, or accident that renders a person unable to perform an activity that would normally be appropriate. Examples would include multiple sclerosis, cerebral palsy, or arthritis. An impairment could be deafness or blindness. Disability relates to the loss of a function that is required for daily activity while impairment refers to a medical condition that causes loss of function.

"Disability Determination" and "Impairment"

In disability determination, the actual capability of an individual to perform a specific task is measured by the amount of capacity actually required to perform the task. This takes into account skills measured by mental capabilities as well as physical capabilities since capacity does not rely on those two measurements alone. Impairment consists of the likelihood that is person is no longer able to function well enough to perform a task for which they had performed in the past. For whatever reason, the person's skills no longer allow them to achieve the same results. It can be a challenge for a physician to confirm an individual's past achievements; however, a comparison could be made from the individual's capabilities to those of an otherwise normal statistical group.

Living with a Disability

For a person suffering from a disability, the disability itself can create problems with the relationships between the individual and his or her friends, family, neighbors, and co-workers. The disability can cause the relationship to be strengthened or to disintegrate. Financial problems from lack of income can also contribute, especially if the non-disabled partner feels increased burden in providing as the sole support. A disabled individual may require assistance to perform even the simplest tasks for daily living such as eating, drinking, dressing, or using bathroom facilities. Although there are services and agencies that can assist with these needs, the extended family members may undergo an adjustment period in seeing the family member in a disabled condition. Therefore, without familial support, the time off from work because of the disability may be extended.

Types of Disabilities

A disability can be in the form of a physical injury to an individual's body such as loss of a limb, loss of sight, hearing loss, quadriplegia, paraplegia, or through an unseen injury such as an internal disease: cancer, AIDS, epilepsy, arthritis, lupus, etc. A second type is a psychiatric disability, such as schizophrenia, depression, mood and/or anxiety disorders, which may have to be treated with medication and, thus coordinating the disability management plan with the individual's physician. A third type of disability relates to behavioral problems. This class may include drug use or alcoholism. Additionally, there are several types of learning disabilities such as Attention Deficit Disorder and dyslexia. Each of these affects the degree to which an individual is able to perform his job.

Disabilities can be the result of an accident, illness, congenital, or injury. Broken down even further, accidents can be the result of a motor vehicle accident, work-site accident, an accident in the home, or an accident out in public such as in a park, playground, shopping mall, or on a city sidewalk. An illness such as AIDS, cancer, or multiple sclerosis can render a person disabled. Additionally, an injury, whether work-related or the result of an accident can also cause a disability. Congenital disabilities are those that are present at birth. Accidents can result in broken bones, torn muscles, loss of limbs, paraplegia, quadriplegia, brain injuries, or spinal injuries. There is no direct correlation between the type of accident and the severity of the injury. Injuries or illnesses can cause the same debilitating factors that can prohibit a person from gainful employment or a productive independent lifestyle. The treatment and the rehabilitation plan should bear similarities to each other; regardless of the way a disability was caused.

Catastrophic Illnesses

In occurrences of illness that are more severely debilitating, the case manager must be sympathetic to the needs and wishes of the individual while keeping costs associated with the medical care and upkeep down. Examples of illnesses that result in higher than normal costs would be AIDS, cancer, head trauma, or spinal cord injuries. While the instances of these illnesses is not as common, their costs can skyrocket considering the prospect of a quick return to work may not be possible. An individual with these types of illness may require specialized care at facilities catering to the specific type of trauma. It is the responsibility of the case manager to negotiate better rates for services if possible and also to closely monitor the types of services received to insure there are no cost overruns. While the case manager is keeping this in mind, he or she also needs to address the needs of the individual and keep their best interests in mind.

Case Management

The traditional definition of case management states that it is the method of coordinating all aspects of an individual's care with respect to social, health, and rehabilitative services while reducing the program's cost and improving one's life and care. The initial steps in case management are to identify those individuals who have recently undergone a disability, then to assess his or her injury and begin planning for treatment, medical benefits, job accommodation, and approximate timeframe for return to work. Services from various agencies and public groups are coordinated depending on the level of care the individual needs. Finally, monitoring of the services and evaluating any care providers is performed. Case management coordination ensures that these services are delivered in a timely manner and in the most cost-effective way.

Disability Case Manager

A disability case manager is the prime advocate for an individual who has been disabled in the workplace. They play a big part in identifying the greatest needs of the disabled person as they plan his or her return to work. Able to assist in a wide variety of areas, the case manager is in the best position to evaluate the level of services received from various agencies to the individual. This centralized attention enables the disabled individual to develop better communication with the case manager and can relay physical and emotional needs which have not been met. The case manager, in turn, can follow up to ensure that no detail is overlooked. This may involve working with outside agencies regarding wages or benefits or even contacting the individual's physician or line supervisor.

Case Manager Selection

A case manager's role is the execution of services in a disability management plan in a timely manner. The person in this position is the central figure in ensuring that all aspects of the plan are followed-through. In selecting this person, it is imperative that they possess advanced skills in the areas in which a company may determine best meets the needs of their industry. For example, if a company has problems with employees returning to work after injuries to the back, then the company may select a rehabilitation counselor or a physical therapist as the main case manager. A company needing help with return to work processes for employees recovering from substance abuse may find that a social worker is best informed on services and programs to meet those needs. In general, a company selects a case manager based on experience and knowledge levels in the fields in which they have the most occurrences of disability.

Case Manager Job Responsibilities

A case manager is selected because of his or her ability to remain organized while dealing with different agencies, departments, and people in managing the care of an individual who is disabled. This person serves to help establish any policies and procedures that would benefit the disabled person and analyzes any data that is collected to determine if corrections need to be made to the policy. Additionally, this person is an advisor to all issues relating to safety and accident prevention in the workplace. The case manager is usually the main point of contact for early intervention of the injury and serves as the liaison between the employee and other key members of the coordinating committee. All of these duties must be performed while keeping in mind that the primary focus should be on helping the disabled person resume a more productive life.

In speaking with an individual for the first time, the case manager may note where the individual would benefit from outside services in addition to his or her regular medical care. These services may be from community agencies that specialize in the types of disabilities that the individual has. A good case manager would have knowledge of these agencies and can make appropriate recommendations to the individual in order to provide a greater level of assistance. During the intake interview, the disabled individual may bring up additional concerns regarding problems with finances, emotional issues due to the disability, and other problems from lack of ability to perform the job as well as before. The case manager should have a list of existing resources to call upon to help the individual with these additional services.

Intake Interview

In the first initial contact with an individual after he or she has agreed to assistance from the disability management program, the case manager sits down and gathers important information regarding his profile and other characteristics. This can include the basic information such as age, gender, marital status, income level, and level of education attained. Detailed history of work including the dates of employment, job responsibilities, title, and day-to-day responsibilities are also included. Other information such as onset of the disability, type of disability, duration of disability, and expected date of recovery, if at all is pertinent to the client's care. The case manager should also be keeping track of all initial and subsequent points of contact with this individual for record-keeping purposes but also to eliminate any confusion down the road. If the individual is covered for medical benefits through Worker's Compensation or private insurance for the injury should be noted. Finally, for those employers whose facility is unionized, the union contact information for the representative should be included.

Rehabilitation

A rehabilitation professional can be in the form of a counselor, mental health professional, occupational or vocational therapist, job placement counselor, or any other health professional who's primary goal is the facilitation of an individual's return to work status as a self-functioning employee. These professionals must coordinate with each other to customize the best plan to meet this goal. Armed with the medical expertise and understanding of chronic illnesses and injuries, they utilize methodology such as evaluations, skills assessments, vocational profiles, and job site visits to determine the skill set of the previous job and determine any potential limitations which need to be followed to increase an individual's potential for success.

Factors that can prohibit a successful return to work for an individual include age since as a person ages, he encounters lack of adaptability in learning a new job or performing more technical tasks. Also, if a pre-existing condition requires new accommodations in the workplace, the individual may require more time in learning to adapt to them. A person's culture and ethnicity can be a factor since there may be instances where education is not as highly valued by the family, for example. The severity of the disability could be another barrier. If the disability prohibits an individual from performing their previous job, then one must allow for vocational retraining or education. Finally, past work history could inhibit a successful return to work if the individual has outdated skills that do not transfer to the current industry.

Rehabilitation Case Analysis

In setting up a case analysis of an individual, one needs to consider all aspects of the person to get a sense of the obstacles and challenges you may encounter during the rehabilitation process. Age is a factor considering that as one grows older, he or she loses the ability to pick up new skills and the learning curve may be greater. Also, the skill level is taken into consideration as the greater the age, more potential for success is placed on those who have higher transferable skills. An unskilled worker will have little or no transferable skills and may be a better candidate for vocational training. Education, therefore, is another aspect to consider in case analysis. The length of schooling, quality of the education or training, and even how long ago the education was obtained is important. Those with high school education and above should have the skills necessary for complex reasoning, abstract thought, and higher language skills. Work history is evaluated also to determine the past levels of physical activity, vocational training, skill levels, and transferability of skills.

Vocational Profile

In a vocational profile, the rehabilitation professional looks for those characteristics that can influence a person's return to work. These are factors that can have either a detrimental or positive affect on the outcome in the disability management plan. Age, educational levels attained, work history, skill levels, and physical exertion requirements of past jobs are all indicators of future vocational plans. Age can determine suitability as newer concepts and skills are picked up more slowly as one ages. A higher educational level attained and also any training received can open doors for more types of jobs. Sporadic work history can make job placements more challenging. Lower skill sets can make it difficult to make a match. Finally, physical abilities to perform one's job may determine whether the new job is sedentary in nature or requiring heavy work.

Planning Return to Work

Initially, a vocational profile is completed allowing the counselor to investigate past work history, skill types, age of client, and determine any transferable skills. Research into the motivation and disability levels of the client is also performed. Familial support of the individual is important as it can assist the client with the help he or she needs to complete treatment and become a more productive member of society. A work site/ job analysis is conducted to see if there are any changes that need to be made to the workstation and the employer is consulted for their input into determining a suitable job environment. Along with these above steps, the counselor needs to also determine the rehabilitation potential of his client.

More often than not, based on the physical exam after the occurrence of an injury, a physician will set a prognosis for the expected recovery time. The physician also would determine the return to work date. Research has shown that this date may not be the best date possible for the disabled individual because it fails to take into account the factors that contributed to the injury. If the employee returns to the worksite too soon and no accommodations or preventative measures have taken place, then there is a higher likelihood for recurrence of the injury. With the supervisor's input and follow-up by the case manager, the employee can be assured that the environment he or she returns is one that takes well being into account. Oftentimes, if the return to work date is open-ended, then it is almost a guarantee that the individual's recovery will be much longer.

Worksite/Job Analysis

In conducting a worksite analysis, one must review the individual's job to identify any barriers to return to work. This may involve pinpointing the need for any reasonable accommodations that need to be made by the employer to ensure that the individual is able to perform the duties of the job without causing undue hardship on the employer. These can range from reduced job responsibilities, revised job descriptions, or assigning new job duties at a lower skill level. For example, for a person with renal disease, an employer would need to rearrange the work required to allow for time off for dialysis. Similarly a person with carpal tunnel syndrome would need an ergonomically designed workspace that inhibits further pain and contributions to symptoms. It can also involve the need to redesign the workspace for wheelchair accommodation or revising the rules to allow for service animals onsite. Educating the employer on the compliance to the Americans with Disabilities Act is also advisable to ensure that the needs of the individual are met.

Common Misconceptions

Common perceptions about a disabled individual who is out on leave is that the person enjoys staying at home and collecting a benefits check. Research has shown that a disabled person is more likely to want to return to work and remain a productive member of the work force. It is important for his or her mental and emotional states to engage in stimulating work and contribute to the financial well being of the household. Additionally, work provides a sense of community and interaction with other adults that staying at home does not provide. Research has also shown how increasing one's disability benefits payments actually increases the amount of time that a person is out from work, whereas, a person with static levels of benefits payments showed no significant increase in the time off.

"Worker's Disability Syndrome"

When a worker loses contact with his or her employer while out on disability leave, the worker tends to feel that the company no longer needs his services. He may express feelings of depression and isolation as a result of his disability. He may lose the motivation to continue with therapy and treatment. His perception of the employer is that the company does not care if he returns or does not even want him back. These people are labeled as "disability dependent". Without sufficient resources such as community agencies or social services to guide him in his return to work, his motivation levels drop and he begins to accept that his disability will define him for the rest of his life. To counteract this attitude, a company or case manager should work with the employee throughout the rehabilitation period from early intervention onward to encourage the healing process back to work.

Employee's Return to Work

Coordinating the care and return to work status of an individual can benefit both the employer and employee. A quick return to work will assist in a faster healing process for the employee who may be anxious to use skills learned in occupational or vocational therapy. The employee may have suffered financial losses as an indirect result of his disability. A faster return would ease up the pressure and worries associated with lack of an income and would increase that individual's earning power. The employer can also see improved production since the employee will have less of a training curve versus a new hire. With the employer's input, a

well thought out disability management plan involves an understanding of the needs of the individual in designing a program that will get him/her back to work in the most efficient manner.

The newly disabled person is dealing with strong emotions related to the disability. These emotions can hinder their return to work by creating barriers in which to overcome their acceptance of their disability. By creating a fast return to work, one can limit the financial burden on the client's family from lack of income, create a better work environment by allowing the client to return to his/her old job in a timely manner, and also avoid much of the "downtime" associated with lack of work. Additionally, you would incur fewer administrative costs in designing a rehabilitation program for the client since fewer resources would be used and medical benefit payouts would be smaller. Also, Social Security Disability income may not have to be tapped. Research has shown that those individuals who are out of work the longest tend not to return and only a small percentage of those who do receive SSDI ever return to work.

Vocational and Rehabilitation Plan Team Approach

For an individual with a disability, the support system in place includes many people devoted to the health and well-being of the individual such as physicians, rehabilitation professionals, vocational counselors, therapists, social workers, and even the patient's own family members. Utilizing the team approach, these people communicate to insure the best plan is formulated to return the individual to work or to a more independent role in society. The physician may make recommendations based on the person's vocational and social history as to the likelihood of rehabilitation. The rehabilitation facility may design an exercise plan based on the notation from the physician on the physical limitations the person may have. Additionally, the family members may help ensure that the patient adheres to the medication schedule as required. Each person in the plan works together to make the transition to work or to an independent lifestyle as smooth as possible.

Holistic Approach

A holistic approach to the case management of a disabled person is best used to ensure that the individual is treated with regards to all aspects of his being. In addition to the immediate task of return to work status, consideration must be taken to these other areas such as spiritual beliefs, cultural or ethnic background, educational background, vocational history, social interactions with friends and family members, acceptance and understanding of the disability, and any psychological and emotional issues as it relates to the disability. These areas can serve as a barrier in the treatment of the individual and can hinder the rehabilitation process. Thoroughly reviewing each of these areas prior to creating a rehabilitation plan can lead to a successful outcome and a positive reentry to work for the individual.

MEDICAL TERMINOLOGY

With the possibility of reading medical charts and physician records to gain a comprehensive understanding of medical diagnosis of an individual in coming up with the rehabilitation plan of a client. There may not be allowable time to research meanings of words and physicians are more readily willing to converse and be more open with a rehabilitation professional who speaks their terminology. Also, in dealing with various members of the health care community such as physicians, therapists, occupational therapists, social workers, nurses, etc., each group may have specialized and unique jargon which may not cross over into other groups. Thirdly, knowledge of medical terminology is to the benefit of the rehabilitation professional, as the client will expect to understand treatment in layman's terms.

MEDICAL ABBREVIATIONS

Abbreviation	Description
b.i.d	twice daily (bis in die)
RA	rheumatoid arthritis
T-2	thoracic vertebrae #2
Hg	hemoglobin or mercury
ESR	erythrocyte sedimentation rate
R.U.Q.	right upper quadrant
TX	treatment

TERMINOLOGY DESCRIBING BODY LANDMARKS

Several common landmark terms are as follows:

Term	Description
Lateral	to the side
Medial	to the center
Posterior	behind the body or relation to the back
Anterior	before or relation to the front
Inferior	below
Superior	above
Prone	laying face downward
Supine	laying face upward

Term	Description
Dorsal	relation to the back
Ventral	relation to the front

Common Origins of Medical Terms

Although the basis of our English words comes from any language, most frequently medical terminology is derived from Latin and Greek. Several examples include "ped", Latin meaning "of the foot" as in pedicure, Greek meaning "child" as in pediatrics. "Brachy", from Greek meaning "short" as in brachycardia. "Plasty" meaning "relating to plastic surgery" as in rhinoplasty is derived from Greek. Another example is "scope"; meaning, "to view or examine with an instrument" as in endoscopy also has Greek origins as does "itis" which means inflammation.

Common Acronyms

Acronym	Description
ADA	Americans with Disabilities Act
IDEA	Individuals with Disabilities Education Act
FHA	Fair Housing Act
ABA	Architectural Barriers Act
ACAA	Air Carriers Access Act

Body Areas Terminology

Term	Description
Carpal	relation to the wrist
Femoral	relation to the thigh
Pelvic	relation to the pelvic girdle
Thoracic	relation to the vertebrae in the upper area of the back
Lumbar	relation to the lower back
Cranial	of or relating to the skull
Abdominal	of or relating to the stomach and intestinal area
Cervical	of or relating to the vertebrae in the neck region
Renal	of or relating to the kidney area

Forms of Income Disability

The three types of wage replacement used by an individual who is not able to return to work are Worker's Compensation, Social Security Disability Insurance (SSDI) and mandatory employer disability programs. Under Worker's Compensation laws, the employer assumes a portion of the financial responsibility for the person who was injured on the job. Although the wages are not equal to the individual's hourly rate, it is commonly around two-thirds of the employee's past rate. Through SSDI, a person with a disability applies for benefits based on his disability rendering himself unable to engage in any substantial gainful activity. This disability must be medically verifiable and consists of a physical or mental impairment lasting twelve months or longer. Additionally, the individual can qualify for benefits if the level of gainful activity is around $500.00 per month. Employer disability programs include long-term disability programs. The amount of benefits under LTD can be reduced depending on whether the individual also qualifies for SSDI benefits.

Worker's Compensation

For the majority of employees injured on the job, the return to work time is minimal, usually in a matter of days. However, there are more severe injuries that take from weeks to months to recover. Longer times out due to an injury results in higher medical costs to the employer and more money spent on Worker's Compensation claims. A proactive system needs to be in place to assess the injury of the worker with a potential to perform light duty at the worksite. Bringing an employee back on a modified schedule or in an accommodated position results in better relations between the employee and employer because of the perception of not losing a valued team member. Additionally, keeping a worker away from the worksite and ceasing communication feeds the notion that the disability is more permanent rather than temporary.

Long-Term Disability

Once it has been determined that an employee is eligible for long-term disability (LTD) based on the injury, it provides for income replacement for up to two years if the employee is unable to perform his or her regular job. LTD also requires that a comprehensive employee assessment is performed on the individual with relation to mental and physical state, concerns of the family, financial needs, past work history, and also the motivational level of the employee on his return to work. Once it has been determined that a return to work is possible, the case manager works with the employee, rehabilitation services, and even Social Security to begin the planning of this process. Long-term disability can incur great costs, however, it is to the advantage of both the employer and employee to facilitate a quick return to work by focusing on the skills the employee has maintained and that which can be accommodated in the workplace.

Early Intervention

In the past, it was more likely that a person injured on the job and out on disability leave would receive no communication from the employer beyond receipt of the disability check. This would lead to feelings of loneliness and isolation, causing the employee to feel as if the workplace had "forgotten" about him. Research shows that there are benefits to early intervention. Initially, a case manager can determine if an employee is receiving the proper medical care to assist the individual towards recovery. Secondly, it is far easier to head off any potential financial problems, for example, with referrals to services that can provide assistance to the individual in the form of Worker's Compensation, SSDI, or other long or short-term disability benefits. Finally, early intervention can change the mindset of an individual who may feel that a return to work may be impossible due to the disability. Showing how an employee is wanted and needed in the old job position is a great motivator in reinforcing the return to work.

Return to Work Incentives

An employee who has been out of work for a period of time has likely suffered from financial difficulties and worry of loss of job status. The purpose of disability management is to return the individual to his former position as quickly as possible. Providing easy access to benefits, medical care, and open communication with the employer is key for a disabled person to focus more on the recovery from the disability. Working with a case manager who can ease the transition back to work by arranging an accommodated work site, possible adjustment to work hours, and unrestricted access to medical care will remove some of the worry associated with being out on disability.

History of Disability

Years ago, a person with a disability could expect to encounter challenges in obtaining suitable work that would accommodate his or her disability. This is especially true if a person had a congenital disability and had difficulty entering the workforce in the first place. Families were advised, in the most severe cases, to institutionalize the person who was affected by the disability. If a person became injured on the job or acquired an illness affecting his or her abilities to perform the duties of the job, the thinking of the times was to gently persuade the person to retire and receive disability benefits. Over time, a new attitude came about in which it was realized the benefits that can be obtained through encouraging and keeping a disabled person in the workforce, both for his benefit as well as that of the employer. Passage of the Americans with Disabilities Act in 1990 ensures that employers cannot discriminate in the workplace those individuals who have a disability.

Disability Legislation

The first type of legislation that affects a disabled person's right to work are laws that force employers to remove policies which prohibit or have excluded a disabled person from obtaining employment or that which limited their opportunities in employment. The second set of laws pertains to allowing a disabled individual access to the types of rehabilitation services that they need to obtain or keep employment. The last set of legislation guarantees that a disabled person receives wage replacement regardless if their injury is temporary or permanent. It generally is not distinguished whether a person received their disability during work or prior to work; however, the intent of this legislation is applied to both scenarios. This ensures that equality is provided to all.

ADA

The Americans with Disabilities Act, signed into law on July 26, 1990, is designed to prohibit any form of discrimination on the basis of an individual's disability. This Act applies to an individual in relation to employment, transportation, use of public buildings and facilities, or communications. Public transportation has been designed to accommodate those with mobility problems. There are methods such as use of TDD or TTY devices allowing for phone communications with the deaf and hard of hearing as well as large print and Braille signs for those with sight disabilities. The ADA stipulates that companies with greater than fifteen employees must comply with the ADA. The ADA is also designed to protect those who, although they have no impairments that prevent employment or performing basic life skills, may have disabilities that cause people to treat them differently. One example would be a person with facial or body scars as can be found on a burn victim.

Medically Related Questions Discrimination

In the hiring process, the company is not practicing discrimination when they ask all the applicants the same set of questions. Only questions related to a measurement of the applicant's skills might be asked. Questions with the intent of screening out individuals with hearing, speaking, reading or writing disabilities are not allowed and prohibited by the guidelines of the ADA. Additionally, questions such as those that ask if a person has ever had a particular illness such as diabetes or cancer are not allowed. The intent behind the questions in the hiring process should be only on whether an applicant is able to perform the duties of the job as to the amount of lifting, sitting, walking, standing, etc. required. More specific medical questions can be asked after a formal offer is extended to a job candidate. However, these cannot be criteria in selecting the final candidate, nor can they be the basis for withdrawing a job offer.

Confidential Information

Confidentiality can be broken down into two distinct categories: relative and absolute. Under relative confidentiality, the information is given out only when it is necessary to disclose the information in order to help the disabled individual. For example, when explaining the reasons for a specific accommodation, the case manager may inform the line supervisor as to the diagnosis of an injury and how the accommodation can help the individual. Beyond that, no other information is given. Absolute confidentiality refers to information that is never to be shared with others. Under protection by law, this information cannot be released unless explicit permission is given so by the individual. Policies and procedures of the disability management plan should clearly outline the company policy in the matter of confidentiality.

Disability Management Confidentiality

While it is necessary to have data collected to determine the effectiveness of a disability management plan, it is important that the confidentiality of the disabled individual is not compromised. The information collected should only be used by those people for whom knowledge of the information is necessary. For example, a case manager working on a file may need access to medical treatment plans in order to coordinate accommodations to a worksite. Drafting the confidentiality agreement and making it available to all key players on the coordinating committee as well as the employees themselves will provide a sense of trust of the employer should a disability occur. Finally, the information collected can be shared on a "need to know" basis rather than openly given to all members of the coordinating committee and in outside organizations. Only that information which is pertinent to each person's role in assisting the disabled individual should be given out. Legally and morally, a company is held to these guidelines.

"Informed Consent"Requirements

With respect to an individual's right to privacy, a company needs to ensure that they are compliant with an individual's desire of limited release of personal information. To comply, the individual must be made aware of each time there is a request of his personal information and he should understand exactly what information will be given out. In addition, knowledge of whom it will be given to such as company name, organization, title, etc. is also helpful. The individual may also want to review the information in writing prior to its release. The individual should also approve or disprove whether the person has the authority to share the information with other parties. Finally, the individual needs to have a complete understanding of any positive or negative outcomes based on this release of the information. To avoid any confusion, the informed consent must be written, dated, and signed with the option to withdraw consent at any time.

"Informed Consent" Confidentiality

A disabled worker, just like any other employee, is entitled to right to privacy of his or her personal data. When an employee is injured on the job, it is important that a policy is in place for effective disability management that does not compromise the trust the employer has placed in his company. Informed consent is simply the permission that the disabled individual has given to release certain parts of his personal information when it pertains to his disability or care. Under informed consent, the individual should be informed as to what information will be disclosed, to whom, for what purpose, and for what time period. At any time, the disabled individual may choose to withdraw his informed consent and no longer release his information. It is important for the company to include the policy on release of information in their disability management plan.

Client Record's Confidentiality

In order to protect the confidentiality of a disabled individual, it is important to maintain proper procedures to ensure that the client's records will not be compromised. To accomplish this, it is the company's responsibility to keep the disability management records separate from other files such as those that pertain to personnel, work history, legal files, and other medical records. Also, client files should not be identifiable by name or social security number, but given a separate identifying number with the master list kept in a separate location. Included in the protection should be all records in the form of tape recordings, videos, and computer files. Also, the individual should have access to his or her own file and be able to make any changes or corrections as they see fit.

Release of Personal Information

For the benefit of an individual, a case manager must consider the positive and negative benefits in releasing private information about an individual. If the request for personal information is made, then the case manager should consult with the individual and go over specifics to the request. The type of information requested as well as for whom and for what purpose should be discussed. The reason for the request and whether it's release would cause any repercussions in the case. Also, questioning whether the release of confidential information would violate any legal policies or ethical standards. Additionally, determining whether the party requesting the information will use it in a responsible manner as the patient's confidentiality is at stake.

Release of Confidential Information Without Permission

In order to completely gain the trust of the disabled individual, care must be taken in the workplace to safeguard the personal information contained in the case management file. If this information is released without permission, the person may be subjected to negative attitudes in the workplace based on what is made known about his or her condition. In addition, the person experiences lack of trust from the employer because the information was released while in their possession. A person could be subjected also to bias from coworkers or supervisors at the workplace and gain a negative reputation. In developing a policy of confidentiality, the company must reinforce the need for privacy on behalf of the individual and also make informed decisions on who is allowed to view the information contained in the files.

Worker Documentation

From the onset, documentation must be written on each point of contact of a person who has been injured or disabled on the job. When they have been deemed as possibly benefiting from assistance through the program, the case manager should log the initial contact on a form. This contact would identify the response of those individuals who either accept or deny assistance through the program. For those that accept, the person is then assigned an appointment time for his or her initial intake interview. At this point the case manager assigns a number to the claimant's file that would not identify him to the particular injury or disability. This is done to protect his right to privacy. The key list that connects these identification number to the real names of the individuals must be kept guarded and under lock and key, accessible only by the case manager and possibly his or her supervisor.

Record-Keeping Form

To keep accurate files in order to monitor the disability management program and also to ensure that all steps are followed in the procedures, the case manager needs to track all points of contact on a record-keeping form. This form could initially identify the individual, date of the injury or diagnosis of the illness, name of the person who referred the individual for assistance, and the expected length of treatment. Additionally, this form could also identify the prognosis of the injury, and whether the person is expected to return to work. Any contact information such as how or when to contact the individual should be included as well. The purpose of recording this information is to accurate track the initial points of contact of a disabled or injured employee regardless of whether they progress into the disability management program.

Findings of Research in Disability Management

In disability management, research has shown that those who have suffered a disability tend to be underemployed or completely unemployed as a result of the disability. For those individuals who do return to work, they face psychological problems as well as those physical problems affecting the manner in which they work. Attitudes from both the workforce and the disabled individual himself can cause a longer period of adjustment in the return to work. Another matter is that the responsiveness of the employer to the needs of the individual can determine the success of the disability management program. Overall, research has shown the cost effectiveness of a formal disability management program reduces payments made out for Worker's Compensation and other long-term benefits. This holds true for both small and large companies, although the size of the organization has a direct effect on its ability to create an effective management program.

Acute and Chronic Pain

Acute pain is severe and lasts only a short while. One example would be the pain encountered with a compound fracture that breaks the skin. Although most people have different levels of pain and the sensitivity to it, acute pain generally warrants a trip to a physician to determine the cause. Chronic pain on the other hand, is longer lasting, more persistent, and is present for some time in response to an injury or illness such as cancer. Acute pain is treated with medication and therapy such as traction or physical therapy to relieve the pain. Acute pain is also localized and specific as to the cause, i.e. the patient is aware of what happened prior to the injury. Physicians may prescribe medication to relieve the pain up to, and including, strong narcotics. With chronic pain, the exact source of the pain may not be known as the radiating pain may be confined to a general area of the body. The duration of chronic pain can be from a few days to months. Treatment involves use of non-narcotic medications, resting the affected area, and moderate activity once the pain subsides.

Chronic Pain

Identifying the specific location of recurring pain and its severity is the first step in building a rehabilitation plan for a person with chronic pain. The duration, initial start of the pain, and any known methods of aggravating the pain will also aid in the development of a suitable rehabilitation plan. Working closely with the physician, other health care professionals or reviewing medical charts, will lead to a higher likelihood of success in returning an individual to a more productive lifestyle. Making note of acceptable physical limitations such as strength, range or motion, loss of sensation of limbs, problems with walking or gait, etc., can help define the rehabilitation plan. The aim of treating chronic pain is to identify factors that diminish the severity of the pain while providing techniques in which to manage pain through possible use of injections, medications, new behaviors learned through occupational or physical therapy, exercise, and relaxation of the affected area.

COPD

Chronic obstructive pulmonary disorders are one of the leading causes of death in the US It is characterized by frequent coughs, production of high amounts of sputum, sneezing, and shortness of breath. Fatigue of the chest muscles utilized in breathing is also present. Illnesses associated with COPD include chronic bronchitis, emphysema, and asthma. Bronchitis is a condition in which the airways of the lungs are inflamed resulting in a cough and heavy production of sputum. Indicators have shown that a common preventable cause of bronchitis is cigarette smoking and exposure to other inhaled pollutants such as dust or fumes from hazardous industries such as mining and paint production. Emphysema is characterized by the expansion, but not the full expulsion of air from the lungs. This can also be caused by cigarette smoking or a rare genetic condition. Asthma is a disease in which the lungs are hyper-reactive to causes such as cold air, exercise, or allergens.

With COPD, an individual experiences a decrease in oxygen flow through the body's systems, most importantly, the lungs. A good rehabilitation program would focus on increasing the lung capacity and also exercise tolerance. In exercise, the individual's performance decreases, as his body cannot tolerate the increase in physical exertion. Oxygen is not flowing throughout the body and the person experiences an increase in heart rate and respiratory distress. Treatment in exercise therapy involves placing the individual on a stationary bicycle or treadmill and allowing them to ease into an increase in amount of time able to complete these exercises. Oxygen supplementation is allowed for severe cases. If performed on a regular basis, the individual finds increased exercise tolerance and ability to perform exercises for a longer period of time. Requiring dedication on the part of the individual to continue with the exercise program, he or she will find, over the course of several months, an increase in respiratory endurance.

In a treatment plan, the most important aspect is prevention. That is, to eliminate or avoid any bronchial irritants. This can include cessation of cigar and cigarette smoking, or avoiding any pollutants that may irritate the bronchial passages. Physicians generally prescribe certain immunizations such as flu shots and pneumonia shots for those suffering from COPD. The belief is that immunizations will decrease the incidence of these illnesses that can exacerbate COPD in those over 60 years of age. Medication for individuals with COPD includes bronchodilators, in the form of an aerosol inhaler, which decreases the sensitivity of the airways and halts bronchospasms. Oxygen is sometimes prescribed for those patients with low oxygen levels and tendency towards pulmonary hypertension. Lung volume reduction surgery and lung transplantation are two additional treatment methods, though not as widely used.

COPD Rehabilitation

An increase in rehabilitation services for a person with COPD has historically resulted in fewer emergency room visits, visits to a physician and also fewer hospitalizations. This is beneficial to the patient as they experience improved social awareness and vocational prospects due to increased mobility. A rehabilitation professional is at the forefront in ensuring the individual's commitment to their rehabilitation program. This can include care programs such as education of the disease for both the patient and his or her family, treatment through the use of bronchodilators, treatment of each bronchial infection as it occurs, and also oxygen therapy, if necessary. Treatment can also consist of breathing techniques and physical therapy in the chest region, social skills, and vocational rehabilitation. Additionally, exercise reconditioning and treatment of right heart failure could also be utilized. By following these steps, the patient is well on his or her way to decreasing the amount of physician visits and can improve the quality of life in living with COPD.

Neuromuscular Disease

In determining the level of activity for a person with neuromuscular disease, it is important to identify the level in which the disease allows the person to function in everyday activities with regards to physical mobility. Secondly, to identify the amount differential between the person's capabilities and the amount of functionality required in doing the work. To determine the person's ability to function, one must take into account the person's age, gender, marital status, education, respiratory impairment, economic circumstances, and social environment of the particular job or occupation. With regards to respiratory function, the ability to perform one's job rests on whether or not the person requires assisted ventilation or an environment free from pollutants that could exacerbate the disease. Additionally, emotional concerns should be reviewed as a potential limitation if the individual has strong signs of anxiety or depression in coping with the disease.

Effect of Neuromuscular Disease on the Respiratory System

In neuromuscular disease, a person experiences difficulties in adequately ventilating their lungs. The weakened muscles render the lungs vulnerable to infections and other complications. They also can interfere with lung capacity. As the disease progresses, the individual can experience increased weakness associated with breathing, malnutrition, muscle weakness, and potentially collapsing of the lungs. The causes of neuromuscular disease can be attributed to anything from spinal muscular atrophies, metabolic, endocrine, hereditary, toxic, vitamin deficiencies, diseases such as botulism, or caused by alcohol or drugs. Treatments can vary, but include resting of the respiratory muscles through assisted ventilation, training of the muscles used in breathing in order to increase endurance and strength, and also better nutrition to provide muscles with the correct ration of carbohydrates, proteins, and fats for better functioning.

Neuromuscular Disease Rehabilitation Potential

Chest rehabilitation is designed to alleviate low oxygen and low carbon dioxide levels in the lungs. This is done primarily through breathing exercises that work the inspiration and expansion of the lungs, as well as diaphragmatic breathing and pursed lip breathing to use during hyperventilation. The goal is to encourage slower, deeper breathing that improves lung expansion and decreases the amount of energy required to breathe. Utilizing rehabilitation exercises to increase breathing can also facilitate a positive outcome for an individual in becoming more independent. While there may always be a need for assisted ventilation, using these physician-prescribed exercises can assist with limiting the muscle fatigue and building endurance in the lung capacity. It is important for a patient not to overdo any physical activity beyond what is most comfortable.

Major Types of Heart Conditions

Congestive heart failure

Coronary artery disease

Cardiomyopathy

Valvular heart disease

Mitral valve prolapse

Hypertension and hypertensive heart disease

Congenital heart disease

Cardiovascular Disease Four Types of Functional Classification

Class I – A patient with diagnosed heart disease who expresses zero symptoms.

Class II – A patient with diagnosed heart disease who expresses symptoms only with moderate physical activity.

Class III – A patient with diagnosed heart disease who expresses symptoms with minimal physical activity.

Class IV – A patient with diagnosed heart disease who expresses symptoms with zero physical activity.

Effects of Cardiovascular Disease

Cardiovascular disease consists of heart strain or progressive failure of the heart muscle to function. It is a leading cause of death in the United States. A timely diagnosis enables the individual to make necessary lifestyle corrections to slow progression of the disease, make surgical corrections to a heart abnormality, and to enlist in rehabilitation services. Increasing the heart's ability to pump blood increases the amount of blood then dispersed to the rest of the body. Gradual lowering the amount of blood in other areas of the body can lead to heart attack, stroke, and other organ damage. Cardiovascular disease can affect a person's ability to perform physical tasks such as lifting or exercising. It can also cause angina or chest pain, and interfere with a person's sense of worth as the disease induces fear of sudden death in some patients.

Effects of Congenital Heart Disease

Although the majority of cases of congenital heart disease are diagnosed and treated early in life, a few people make it through to adulthood without having prior knowledge of the disease. In either case, a prompt response, usually aggressive surgical procedures are performed to lessen the severity of the disease and improve cardiovascular function. An adult who is newly diagnosed with the disease can expect a quick medical intervention to correct the abnormality. An assessment will be made on any ongoing functional limitations in terms of job capabilities and work restrictions. A rehabilitation counselor would need to be retained to explain to the individual how to function in life with this new diagnosis and assist the person on the road to recovery.

Cardiovascular Disease Five Types of Therapeutic Classification

Class A – The patient does not require any physical limitations to activity.

Class B – The patient does not require limitations to normal activity; however, severe activity should be restricted.

Class C – The patient requires moderate limitations to normal activity.

Class D – The patient requires high limitations on normal activity.

Class E – The patient requires complete bed rest or rest in a chair.

Hypertension

Hypertension is known to be a "silent killer" since its occurrence does not usually involve a presentation of symptoms. A diagnosis is usually made after symptoms develop through other complications such as coronary artery disease and vascular disease. Hypertension can also cause vague non-specific complaints such as fatigue, headache, blurred vision, or weakness. A thorough examination of the individual's heart, vision, kidneys, and cerebral vascular system is performed that will indicate cellular changes leaning towards hypertension. Chest x-rays, stress tests, EKG's and echocardiograms are specific tests used in the diagnosis. Complications that arise from hypertension include renal failure, higher incidence of stroke or heart attacks, and congestive heart failure. Pain in the lower extremities can occur due to the decrease in blood flow to these parts of the body. Transient ischemic attacks can affect the blood flow to the brain. In evaluating one's blood pressure, higher systolic and diastolic numbers reveal increased pressure on the heart to pump blood. Blood pressure is identified as a ratio between systole and diastole represented as systolic/diastolic. A reading of 120/80 is considered normal. Systolic refers to the amount of pressure when the heart is contracting blood out of the heart chambers. Diastolic refers to the reading when the heart muscle is at rest. Therefore, hypertension is defined as a systolic reading greater than 140. Its causes can be related to hereditary, vascular abnormalities, kidney disease, and abnormalities in the endocrine system. Increases in stress can also play a role. Genetically, higher blood pressure levels are related to an increase in heart disease.

Depending on the level of severity of the hypertension and the degree to which other organs may be affected, a rehabilitation counselor can expect to see a wide variety of functionality in these individuals. Those individuals who were diagnosed with hypertension after a diagnosis of kidney failure, for example, may need greater assistance with vocational rehabilitation than another individual for whom very few changes need to be made. The level of activity can also differ depending on how well the person responds to treatment. A physician recommendation is necessary in these cases as to the degree of activity level based on the medical treatments the person is expected to follow in order to avoid any additional damage to the heart muscle. In spite of a diagnosis of hypertension, the majority of individuals who follow the prescribed treatment plan can expect to lead a productive life in terms of work, leisure activities, and lifestyle.

Coronary Artery Disease

With coronary artery disease being the leading cause of death in the United States, it is imperative to understand the risk factors leading to this diagnosis. Hypertension, high cholesterol levels, obesity, lack of exercise, diabetes, stress, and smoking are all causes that contribute to the development of this disease. Along with high cholesterol levels comes the buildup of plaque in the blood stream that decreases the amount of blood that can easily pass through the blood vessels. Nicotine also contributes to this decrease in blood flow through constricting of blood vessels during the act of smoking. With coronary artery disease, a decreased amount of oxygen is making it from the blood vessels to the heart muscle. Angina appears along with arrhythmia and ventricular fibrillation. With the decrease in oxygen, a myocardial infarction occurs causing the affected portion to die. With the inefficiency of the heart muscle to transport oxygen, fluids do not flow causing congestion and creating a life-threatening emergency. Major signs of coronary artery disease include:

- Angina pectoris– Refers to chest pain.
- Myocardial infarction – Occurs when blood supply to the heart is interrupted. Also called a heart attack.
- Arrhythmia – A disorder causing the heart to beat in an irregular pattern.
- Congestive Heart Failure – A condition in which the heart does not pump enough blood through to the organs causing edema, fluid in the lungs, fatigue, and shortness of breath.

Review Video: Coronary Artery Disease
Visit mometrix.com/academy and enter code: 950720

Coronary Artery Disease Treatment Plan

In developing a plan of rehabilitation for a person with a cardiovascular disease, it is important to note the level of activity prescribed by the physician. Most individuals can attain a degree of light duty at work. Heavy lifting and carrying is usually restricted, however, moderate activity is beneficial to exercising the heart muscle back to health. The possibility of angina is great and often the patient remains on medication to alleviate this. When it does occur, cessation of the activity that caused it is usually recommended. Additionally, vocation rehabilitation is necessary to determine if the person is able to return to work in his or her former capacity. A lighter duty position may be required that does not cause undue stress on the individual. The rehabilitation professional must also take into account a person's emotional well being as the reality of living with a serious disease may make the person fearful of any activity and depression and anxiety may set in as they are dealing with possibility of his or her mortality.

Cardiovascular Disease Rehabilitation Potential

The potential for rehabilitation is greatest for an individual whose cardiovascular disease may not be as severe. Keeping to the treatment and exercise plan as prescribed by the physician and making the necessary work modifications can lead to a successful return to work. Through education of the causes of the disease as well as elimination of some of the risk factors, for example, high cholesterol and smoking, an individual can expect to return to a more independent way of life. By working with the person's employer to develop job modifications, the rehabilitation counselor can ease the person back into the mindset of work, thereby dispelling the notion that the individual is not physically capable of returning to work and encouraging him towards a positive, rather than negative, frame of mind.

Loss of Hand Functions

With approximately one-third of all workplace injuries involving injuries to the hand and upper extremities, it is important to note how this disability affects an individual. The hand serves multiple functions in that it is used to write, shake hands with others, grasps objects, opens doors, assists with dressing and feeding one's self, and lifting objects. With the loss of these functions, an individual must learn to use the non-injured hand in a greater capacity or retrain the injured hand by making adaptations. The hand contains a great deal of sensory nerves, and it allows an individual to "read" certain objects simply by how they feel in the hand. Additionally, a greater proportion of the cerebral cortex area of the brain is used towards interpreting nerves from the hand. The only greater portion is reserved for the lips and face. Therefore, a person who loses function in the hand loses not only ability to grasp, but also part of the sense of touch.

Hand Injury Functional Limitations

A fingertip injury is one of the most common hand injuries sustained at work in a manufacturing facility. Depending on the degree to which the injury occurs in proximity to the joint, the patient sustains some loss of grip strength as well as manual dexterity. In cases where the majority of the finger was lost, job retraining may be necessary. In addition, the higher number of digits affected will significantly increase the lack of function of the hand overall. Through research, a thumb provides 40% of hand function, the middle and ring finger provides 20% each, and the index and pinky provide 10% each of the overall function. Other common injuries to the hand in the workplace are fractures, wrist injuries and carpal tunnel syndrome. Fractures are easiest to rehabilitate from and the time off to recover can be measured in weeks. Carpal tunnel syndrome is a compression injury affecting the nerves at the base of the hand. Rest, medication, steroid shots, an ultimately surgery is required if the symptoms do not improve.

Injuries That Cause Loss of Hand Function

An injury occurring to the hand can originate from many sources: burns, tears, fractures, nerve damage, torn ligaments, or ruptured tendons. For minor lacerations and burns, a simple bandage may do, but in more severe cases, sutures and skin grafts may be necessary. Fractures require immobilization and casting while torn ligaments and tendons require surgery. Along with these treatments, therapy needs to be initiated to restore function to the hand and increase range of motion and strength. In evaluating the patient with a hand injury, it should be noted whether or not the injury occurred in the dominant hand since, during recuperation, the patient may need to be retrained in common skills such as using utensils with the non dominant hand.

Hand Injury Recovery

In returning the individual's hand to one of strength, endurance, and mobility, the rehabilitation professional should consider several of the following activities. Exercising the hand and gradually adding additional weights or repetitions builds strength. Using the hand in the practice of daily activities of living such as writing, opening doors, or grasping objects can also build strength. Practicing these skills can shorten the time needed for rehabilitation. The therapist should also consider training of the non-dominant hand if it was the one not injured to give the individual greater independence while the injured hand heals. Most importantly, the motivation level and the attitude of the individual will make a difference in how well he responds to therapy and treatment.

Orthotics and Prosthetics

An amputation involves the partial loss or total loss of one part of the body. For those disabled individuals, a rehabilitation plan consists of a fitting of either a prosthetic or orthotic. A prosthetic consists of a device that is designed to replace the missing limb. Most commonly known as an artificial limb, it can be either an artificial arm or leg. Its purpose is to provide the individual with the tools necessary to regain range of motion or grasp. It is customized to fit the individual perfectly to his or her body shape yet is only fitted after the person reaches a level of thickness in the skin of the affected body part, and edema has decreased in the remaining limb. An orthotic is commonly referred to as a brace that is designed to support or stabilize the affected part of the body.

Assistive Devices

In addition to the devices used to stabilize the affected limbs, neck, or back of an individual, a rehabilitation profession has at his disposal various other assistive devices that are used to make daily functions easier to manage. One such tool is the use of canes, crutches, or walkers to assist in movement such as walking. These tools help maintain the independence of the individual and allow the person to rely less on others for assistance with ambulation. To assist those with their grasp, devices such as a tool for extended reaches, long handled grippers, and specially designed computer keyboards are available. Additionally, mouthpieces to assist a quadriplegic individual with pushing buttons on a telephone or keyboard are also available. Finally, customizable wheelchairs can allow greater independence of a disabled individual.

CATEGORIES OF ORTHOSES

Category	Description
AFO	Ankle Foot Orthosis
KAFO	Knee Ankle Foot Orthosis
HKAFO	Hip Knee Ankle Foot Orthosis
WHO	Wrist Hand Orthosis
WDWHO	Wrist-Driven Wrist Hand Orthosis
SEO	Shoulder Elbow Orthosis
LSO	Lumbosacral Orthosis
TLSO	Thoraco Lumbo Sacral Orthosis
CTLSO	Cervical Thoraco Lumbo Sacral Orthosis

DIABETES LEADING CAUSE OF AMPUTATION IN THE UNITED STATES

Diabetes can affect other parts of the body through changes in the levels of glucose in the blood. The body does not have the sufficient means necessary to either produce insulin or to process the amount of insulin made in response to caloric intake. Over time, this imbalance can affect the eyes, heart, kidneys, nerves and circulatory system. With an injury to the extremities, in particular the feet, infection may set in and healing can be slow. The extremity may die due to the lack of sufficient blood circulation. When it reaches this point, the only alternative is an amputation. Depending on the degree to which the tissues of the affected body part have died determines the location of the amputation. Diabetes that is well controlled does not usually result in amputation.

AMPUTATION CAUSES EMOTIONAL CHANGES

Research has shown that after surgery in which a person's body part was amputated, the person would begin the healing process much faster when a prosthetic part was bandaged along with the amputated limb. The person may undergo emotional stages that are similar to those of the stages of death and dying. Easing the transition by allowing the person to gradually come to terms with the loss of a limb can help with the initial adjustment period. Grief and a sense of loss for the affected limb is common as is sadness over the loss of the activities that the patient may feel he or she is no longer able to do. Anger, especially if the amputation was the result of an accident versus an illness such as foot problems resulting from diabetes. Finally, acceptance as the person realizes the extent of the amputation and the motivation to forward with life and normal activities.

Amputation Complications

At the actual site of the amputation, the individual may feel "phantom pain" from the onset that may require medication in dealing with this chronic pain. Additionally, there is a risk of infection at the amputation site post-surgery that can also be treated with antibiotics. Contractures may develop through lack of use of the affected limb either before or after the surgery. Edema may be present and while this may hinder correct fitting of prosthesis, a prosthetic device may help decrease the amount of swelling in that area. Also, skin ulcerations may occur due to a poor-fitting prosthesis, lack of cleanliness around the prosthesis, an infection, or where the prosthesis rubs against the skin.

Neurology

Neurology is the branch of medicine that deals with nervous system disorders. These may include illnesses or injuries associated with the central nervous system, the peripheral nervous system, and the autonomic nervous system. Occasionally, neurologists deal with conditions related to the musculoskeletal system. The list of conditions that neurologists see can include epilepsy, migraines, seizures, sleep disorders, cerebral palsy, infections such as encephalitis and meningitis, Parkinson's disease, Tourette's syndrome, multiple sclerosis, tumors of the spinal cord, and traumatic injuries to the brain or spinal cord. This list is not all-inclusive. Neurologists may focus their education on a specialized area such as movement disorders, epilepsies, demyelinating diseases, genetic disorders, or spinal cord disorders.

Usually with a referral from a physician, the patient comes to the neurologist with a set of symptoms that require further examination as to the cause. The neurologist will initially obtain the patient's history then move on to the physical examination. This portion of the examination is in greater detail to include the person's mental state. Tests that review the person's reasoning ability, memory, speech, and ability to solve arithmetic problems are covered. Tests reviewing the function of the cranial nerve are also given to measure any abnormalities in facial nerves, sight, and sense of smell. The person's gait is measured to detect any abnormalities in walking. Cerebral function is measured for any abnormalities in the person's movement and coordination. Finally, motor and sensory skills are measured before the neurologist reviews the data to determine any additional laboratory and imagining tests. Only after all this is completed will the neurologist make a definitive diagnosis and offer options for treatment.

Neurological Disorder

Diseases of the central nervous system are classified into two groups: nonprogressive and progressive. A nonprogressive disease is one that does not worsen with time. Aside from the initial onset of the disease, the patient can be expected to make adjustments to his personal and work lifestyle to accommodate the disability. One such example would be a stroke victim. Long-term goal setting usually works towards returning the person to the quality of life they experienced prior and making the necessary vocational adjustments. For a person with a progressive disease such as multiple sclerosis or a brain tumor, there is little chance of improvement as the years pass and the person may experience an ongoing increase in symptoms. With these cases, focus is geared on treatment of the disability and not as much on retraining an individual for the workforce as the boundaries of the disease may make its futile effort.

EPILEPSY

Epilepsy is described as a disability marked by a variety of conditions that end in seizures. A seizure is a state in which the brain's electrical activity is in a mode of chaos resulting in excessive electrical discharges causing temporary loss of bodily control of the limbs and torso. Seizures can emanate from one portion of the brain, called a partial seizure, or from both cerebral hemispheres, called a generalized seizure. Seizures may occur without warning and can last from a few seconds to a few minutes. The etiology of seizures lies in a brain injury, infection, vascular disease, birth trauma, genetics, or is related to a substance abuse problem. Epilepsy is classified as a chronic disorder in which there are no known indicators of factors that initiate a seizure.

EPILEPSY TREATMENT

Several treatment options are available for a person with epilepsy. These can include medication specific to the type of seizures that are experienced. Initially hospitalization is required when one first experiences seizures to determine the cause, however, outpatient services are recommended if the seizures occurred some time prior to being seen by the physician. Prescription medications for epilepsy are based on the specific type of seizure experienced by the individual. Classified as primary and secondary drugs, physicians try one after another to come up with a medication that results in well-controlled epilepsy. Too high of a dosage of one drug can result in toxic levels of the medication within the person's bloodstream. An additional method of treatment involves surgery on the portion of the brain where lesions or tumors are present. Removal of these lesions decreases the likelihood of tumors from recurring, however, this option is only recommended if medications have failed due to the high incidence of lasting serious side effects.

EPILEPSY AND VOCATION

For an individual with epilepsy, a choice of a career is a challenging one in which a person needs to weigh the severity of the condition with that of obtaining suitable work that does not put either himself or others in harm's way. Some physicians may even put driving restrictions on an individual with severe or uncontrollable seizures. The vocational counselor must be aware of several factors in order to suggest a course of action towards obtaining suitable employment. These can include the type and severity of the seizures, the duration of the seizures and how long it takes for the person to recover, and the also whether the individual has any advance warnings prior to a seizure. Additionally, it is helpful to know if there is loss of consciousness during a seizure, whether any precipitating factors such as flashing lights are likely to cause a seizure, and also what medications are necessary to decrease the frequency of the seizures.

Traumatic and Atraumatic Brain Injuries

A traumatic injury is one that results from an outside force to the brain that causes changes in the individual's cognitive, physical, and psychosocial aspects of his being. This injury can be the result of open head or closed head injuries. A closed head injury is usually diagnosed through an MRI or CT scan. Loss of consciousness, loss of memory, confusion, and disorientation can result from closed head injury. An open head injury is easier to diagnose, as damage to the exterior of a person's head is readily visible. Generally resulting from a stabbing or gunshot wound, the person may or may not experience a coma at the initial onset; however, a physician may order a medically induced coma to aid in healing. An atraumatic brain injury is one where the injury occurs due to malformations in the arteries and veins present in the brain, strokes, and aneurysms. Tumors, lack of oxygen, and meningitis are all examples of an atraumatic brain injury.

Causes of Traumatic Brain Injury (TBI)

The cause of traumatic brain injury can be attributed to car accidents, boating accidents, strokes, infections, falls, shooting injuries, brain aneurysms, or stabbings. Defined, TBI is an external force from outside the body that causes significant loss of cognitive and reasoning abilities, memory loss, and lack of coordination of the physical body. Psychosocial changes occur which can lead to depression, personality changes, frustration, and possibly substance abuse. The most commonly affected demographic appears to be young males from ages 14-24, then infants, and finally the elderly. The majority of TBI's, or traumatic head injuries, are caused by vehicular accidents. Alcohol usually plays a strong role in the occurrence of TBI's. A large percentage of people with TBI's were intoxicated at the time of injury. Traumatic brain injuries can either be classified as closed head, or open head injuries.

TBI Individual Rehabilitation

Depending upon the severity of the injury, the person with TBI can experience a short rehabilitation period or the person may never return to the physical and mental state he or she had prior to the accident. Physical therapy is utilized to assist with the need for learning to walk again, a side effect of being in a comatose state. Utilizing first a wheelchair, then a walker, cane, and finally able to mobilize unassisted, a person can regain control of their walking in a matter of weeks or even months. Speech therapy and language therapy are used to retrain the person to use their speech muscles in forming sounds. Occupational therapy is used to assist with relearning simple life skills such as putting on clothing, tying shoes, or using utensils while eating. Finally, cognitive therapy is important in that it teaches the person to use memory skills and other undamaged parts of the brain to assist with everyday tasks.

Basic Anatomy of the Back

The posterior area of the human body consists of the spinal canal, vertebrae, and discs. The spinal canal protects the nerves running the length of the body. The discs, consisting of a soft gelatinous substance, gradually harden over decades and by middle age, tend to become more fibrous and brittle. The chance of injury is increased, and the person experiences a decrease in height due to the settling of the discs. The vertebrae then begin to settle and may not remain in alignment that can also cause pain with or without activity. The spinal canal protects the spinal cord and nerves. These nerve and associated ligaments provide the degree of movement and flexibility, greatest in the early years.

Back or Neck Pain

Individuals who have been injured on the job may be looking for a financial windfall if they seek litigation for their claim. These people may unintentionally set themselves up to delay the rehabilitation process or amplify the amount of pain they are experiencing. This may be especially true if the person did not like his or her job or the supervisor. Additional factors that cause a slower return to work would be poor physical state prior to and after the injury, smoking or excessive physical activity that exacerbates the pain. Most people experience anxiety and concern and if the person is overwhelmed with financial matters or whether they will be able to return to work, the stress may be compounded. Finally, adherence to the set prescribed medications and physical therapy plan plays a role in determining the duration of time off recovering from the injury.

With the large numbers of nerves radiating from the spinal canal to other areas of the body, the pain can thus radiate from one part of the back down the arms or legs for example. The pain is not always localized, but can shoot either upwards or downwards from the point of origin. The vertebral discs are a common source of pain for those over the age of 30, but other causes can include sprains, strains, tears, or even arthritis. Additionally, muscles, tendons, and ligaments can also be a source of back pain. A herniated disc can cause pain in which settling occurs and bones then rub against one another. Another serious form of pain is called sciatica, which involves radiating pain down the leg. Sciatica or other nerve damage can result in loss of feeling, muscle weakness or even paralysis.

Back Injury Rehabilitation

Some individuals who are able to return to his or her previous job with accommodations may find it challenging as the level of job satisfaction plays a role in how quickly the person recovers. With increasing age, it is more difficult to return to the same youthful activity level as degeneration of the spinal canal has occurred. Loss of flexibility and resilience in the back causes additional pain and lack of mobility. Adhering to physical therapy and prescribed medications can assist with maintaining one's role in the workforce; however, motivation is a strong factor in the decision to return to work. Education on preventative measures and adaptation of safety devices can promote healing and prevent future injuries. The sooner the individual returns to work, the better his chances of remaining a productive member of the workforce. Research has shown that the increased amount of time off to recover delays the return to work, sometimes permanently.

Spinal Cord Injury (SCI)

Although a SCI is generally known to cause the inability to walk or move one's arms, additional bodily functions can be affected. Lack of bladder and bowel control can occur if the person no longer has the sensation of when to void. Sexual function can be impaired and the person may need to rely on medication or artificial stimulation to maintain intimacy with his or her partner. Although a female may become pregnant, lack of sensation may cause problems when undergoing labor. Men may have to resort to artificial insemination as the levels of sperm may drop. Breathing may become difficult as the person may require ventilation to assist with breathing when weak chest muscles no longer perform the job. Finally, susceptibility to infections can increase due to lack of mobility. This can include pressure sores or pneumonia.

Conductive Versus Sensorineural Hearing Loss

Conductive hearing loss is defined loss of hearing as a result of damage to the outer or middle ear. This damage interferes with the transmission of sound waves to the cochlea. Hearing loss to this degree can be a result of genetics, injury, blockage, or other damage. Treatment involves removal of blockage, use of hearing aids, and surgery in certain cases. Sensorineural hearing loss results from damage to the auditory system which includes nerve damage to the inner ear, auditory nerve, or injury to the part of the brain relating to hearing. Hearing aids may or may not have any effect because in this type of hearing loss, sound may get through however, the pitch and spoken word is distorted. Causes can include maternal illness, high fever, head injuries or tumors. Treatment methods vary to include hearing aids, cochlear implants, and also educating the individual in lip-reading.

Visually Impairment

Blindness and vision loss results in increased capabilities of the other senses. In reviewing a client's return to work status, one needs to review the adaptability of these skills in a work environment. Various levels of blindness are better suited for some jobs than others. The rehabilitation counselor must define the skill set the client is best suited for, whether use of aids is warranted depending on severity of vision loss, what degree of mobility one has, and the level in which they have gained in previous training, employment or education. Defining skill sets that use the remaining amounts of vision is key in enabling the individual to maintain certain levels of self-esteem and independence.

Type II Diabetes

Research has proven that maintenance of ideal body weight in relation to a person's height is a factor that can prevent the onset of diabetes. Healthy diets consisting of a balance between meats, fruits, vegetables, dairy products, and breads will ensure that blood glucose levels will remain at acceptable levels in the body and not allow for spikes that can signify an impaired glucose tolerance. A diabetic counselor or nutritionist will determine, using an individual's profile, the correct amounts of food and meal times best suited to maintain healthy glucose levels. Along with maintaining a proper diet, regular exercise on a weekly basis will keep a person's weight in proportion to height and thus help ward off advent of diabetes. Regular monitoring of blood glucose levels for a person of an at-risk race will pinpoint any abnormalities that may signal further testing.

Type II diabetes is also referred to as non-insulin dependent diabetes. Several factors can be identified as the cause of this disease, which is characterized by insulin resistance, or low levels of insulin produced by the pancreas. The body uses insulin to metabolize glucose in the blood. Getting the body's glucose levels under control is the main concern to head off additional severe health problems. One way to do this is to regulate glucose levels in the blood through maintaining a healthy weight. A person's age as well as genetic makeup including race also play a role in potential development in this disease. With the steadily rising numbers of obese individuals, there also has been an increase in the numbers of newly diagnosed diabetics. Statistically, persons of the following races have a higher disposition towards the disease: African American, Mexican American, and Native Americans.

Complications of Diabetes

Uncontrolled or poorly managed diabetes can lead to complications in other parts of the body. Narrowing of the arteries in the lower extremities, foot ulcers, infection and gangrene in the lower limbs could eventually lead to amputation if these conditions are left unchecked. Nerve damage, known as neuropathy, can occur throughout the body, resulting in tingling sensations in the extremities, again, most commonly in the lower extremities. If untreated, can also lead to loss of sensation and traumatic injuries, as the individual may be unaware of any damage that occurs to that part of the body. Hemorrhaging and weakness of the retinas of the eyes is called retinopathy. Severe retinopathy can lead to blindness. Additionally, renal failure, sometimes requiring dialysis or a kidney transplant, can develop due to diabetic nephropathy. This term refers to the lack of protein in the urine and the build up of waste products in the blood stream. Keeping diabetes well managed and blood sugar levels under control can minimize these complications.

Hemophilia

This hereditary disease is defined as an inability to coagulate blood in response to an injury. Out of the 13 known coagulant factors, researched have pinpointed factor VIII or factor IX as the cause for this disease. Contrary to popular belief, a hemophiliac is not considered a "bleeder" in the sense that profuse amounts of blood comes forth upon the slightest cut, but rather, the person has a marked decrease in the body's ability to coagulate (or clot) blood. This disability manifests itself in all aspects of the body. In addition to the bleeding as a result of a skin lesion, joints, muscles, and even the brain is subject to bleeding. Frequency of bleeding is a strong consideration. Although hemophiliacs are not weak individuals with delicate dispositions, it must be taken into consideration the type of employment the individual can do which will not exacerbate the disability. When bleeding does occur, aside from a skin lesion, it most commonly affects the body in this order: knees, elbows, ankles, shoulders, hips, and wrists. Over a period of time, joint damage due to the hemophilia can occur.

Rheumatic Disease

A rheumatic disease is one that affects the joints and connective tissues of the skin, bones, or muscles. These diseases can include rheumatoid arthritis, osteoarthritis, gout or lupus, to name a few. A less common rheumatic disease is scleroderma. While osteoarthritis is the most common disease, rheumatoid arthritis has the higher disability rate. These diseases render an individual with localized swelling in the joints, pain, and loss of functionality. Deformities can also exist. Although these diseases have no cure at this time, the treatment plan could involve medication, surgery or joint replacement. As the disease progresses, more accommodations need to be made to account for loss of movement, loss of strength, and possibly difficulties with standing and walking.

Genetic Counseling

For an individual who has been diagnosed with a disease whose etiology is hereditary, it is sometimes warranted that they undergo genetic counseling if they are concerned about passing the disease along to their offspring. Genetic counseling's sole existence is due to making an informed decision on whether to reproduce. The goals of genetic counseling include obtaining a complete understanding of the disease and the risk levels for future generations, understanding the probable causes of the disease and the resources that may become available and dealing with the decision to reproduce after all the information on the disease has been obtained. Prenatal testing for genetic disorders is done usually through amniocentesis or DNA testing. The decision on whether to continue with a pregnancy after the embryo has been determined to have a genetic disorder is not an easy one.

Genetic Counseling for a Couple

The counselor, with medical knowledge and the ability to explain in lay terms the pros and cons of continuing with a pregnancy after genetic testing, needs to be sympathetic to the couple's emotions. Feelings of loss, hope, fear, frustration, and anger are common emotions as the couple comes to terms with the reality of the pregnancy. The role of the counselor is not to provide his own personal opinion, but to support the decision made by the couple. Addressing the couple's needs and dealing with the issues while establishing rapport would increase the lines of communication and allow the counselor to be responsive to the family and allow them to come to terms of ending the pregnancy or dealing with the reality of raising a special needs child.

Genetic Counseling Information Abused

As genetic testing becomes more cost efficient and easy to obtain, the information garnered from the tests could be used in a manner to discriminate against individuals for a perceived, although not actual, disability. At the forefront could be an employer biased against a person with a certain disability or an insurance company who could deny selling a life insurance policy for the potential a person has in developing a "costly" disease. Additionally, insurance companies may consider cutting back on the benefits payments if they discover the person was aware of his genetic tendency towards a specific disorder. It is possible that employers, educators, law enforcement officials, and others could use information gathered through genetic testing in a negative matter without fully understanding the potential disruption their use may cause.

Role of a Rehabilitation Counselor in Genetic Counseling

A rehabilitation counselor has experience in dealing with community agencies that can provide services geared towards special needs children. This experience can be beneficial to a couple that is considering continuing with a pregnancy after discovering a genetic disorder. In addition to providing support, the rehabilitation counselor can also advocate on behalf of the unborn child by discussing issues with the parents on potential discrimination challenges that their child may face. He can also inform them on any legal rights their child may have. The rehabilitation counselor can also put the new family in touch with others who have gone through the same scenario as a mentoring learning experience. Additionally, serving as a technical advisor, the counselor can paint a portrait of day-to-day life with a special needs child to acclimate the parents and other family members with the new responsibilities they will face.

Sexuality

Sexuality deals with how we feel about ourselves, how we relate to others, and to our immediate surroundings. Sexuality at its basic level is the expression of our physical urges. Sexuality involves both physical and psychological aspects: physical in terms of our innate urges and psychological for our need to connect with others emotionally, affectionately, and through other expressions of love. From the standpoint of the disabled individual, their sexuality is as much a given right as it is to the non-disabled person. Unfortunately, society tends to treat a disabled person as a non-sexual being. Through communication with the disabled individual, the counselor should ensure that this aspect of the rehabilitation plan is covered.

HIV, AIDS, CDC

HIV – Human Immunodeficiency Virus – Virus that breaks down the body's immune system. This virus is the main causative factor of AIDS.

AIDS – Acquired Immunodeficiency Syndrome – A highly contagious incurable disease in which the body loses its ability to fight off infection and viruses.

CDC – Centers for Disease Control – Part of the US Public Health Service whose focus is on monitoring and tracking the spread of diseases.

Modes of HIV Transmission

Human immunodeficiency virus (HIV) can be transmitted through bodily fluids contained in white blood cells, vaginal and seminal secretions via sexual contact. Additionally, it is also transmitted through various methods of blood transfusions. During a medical or surgical procedure, it is sometimes called upon for units of whole blood to be transfused into another patient. If this blood has not undergone HIV testing, then the patient runs the risk of contracting the virus. Hemophiliacs have also been known to acquire HIV through acquisition of whole blood products in treating their disease. With blood products being tested prior to use on transfusions, this form of transmission is being reduced. IV drug users who share common needles and syringes are at risk since minute amounts of blood may still be present on the needle. An HIV positive mother could pass the virus to her unborn child during delivery. Also, despite precautions, health care workers are at risk in the event that a needle, used to draw blood, for example, accidentally pierces the skin of the worker who, therefore, has the potential for developing the virus. New advances are being made to reduce risks associated with health care workers administering shots or drawing blood from HIV infected individuals.

HIV Positive Rehabilitation

In determining the rehabilitation potential the counselor must look first to the degree in which the HIV virus has affected the person's individual health. Individuals who have greater degrees of immunodeficiency have less likelihood in maintaining the ability to return to work. The age is also a factor because the younger one is, the more likely he would have greater amounts of strength, agility, and stamina, which lends himself to more energy available to work. Also a factor is that a person with HIV generally lacks any physical disabilities such as lack of appendage, spinal cord injuries, confinement to a wheelchair, allowing for the potential to hold employment at a level of light to medium duty work.

Plastic Surgery

Plastic surgery is defined as the application of processes by which a surgeon utilizes his skills to repair or correct wounds in the body and face. These wounds can be the result of injury, illness, or accidents that create a disability for the individual. A large percentage of plastic surgery performed is of a cosmetic nature. Although physical appearance does not encompass all of a person's being, it stands true that an improved appearance heightens the degree of an individual's self-esteem, an important aspect in the rehabilitation process. Additionally, with the increased function of the repaired area, the individual gains confidence and mobility which otherwise would be lacking. This leads to a greater potential for return to work.

Arms and Hands Burn Injuries

The counselor needs to first look at any physical limitations that may be present. These limitations can affect ability to grasp, pinch, lift, carry objects, and write. It there is an amputation of finger appendages, the individual must be taught alternative methods of coordination and manual dexterity usually through occupational therapy. Scar tissue can also decrease the range of motion capabilities and physical activity. Emotionally, the counselor should be aware of the degree to which the individual has come to accept his/her disability. Severity of the disability is often not a good indicator. In some cases, a smaller disfigurement has a greater psychological impact than a person who may have a more noticeable or severe disability. Counselors need to be sensitive to this issue when evaluating a client's case.

Learning Disabilities

A person with a LD exhibits problems in several critical areas such as language, mathematics, study skills, and attention span. Difficulties in language skills manifest in poor perception of sounds, lack of ability in recognizing syllables in words, mispronunciation of words, inability to read well, and poor penmanship. Mathematical skills may be lacking as well resulting in inability to understand basic mathematic concepts, and inability to solve more complex problems. Poor study and organizational skills and lack of focus are examples of how difficult it may be for a LD individual to perform these tasks. These challenges can affect the ability to function in society unless the person has been trained with coping mechanisms that allow him to learn new methods of functioning.

With as much as 15% of the population affected by a learning disability, tests are continually developed to determine the extent of the disability. This type of a disability can result in lifelong consequences as it relates to interpersonal relationships, ability to obtain and hold employment, and ability to lead a productive independent life. A learning disability is defined as a disorder that leads to reduced capabilities in reasoning, perception, understanding verbal and written concepts, memory, communication, social functioning, coordination, and poor maturity levels. A person with this disability may have it as a result of another condition such as Down's syndrome. In order to successfully diagnose this condition, a series of tests must be conducted on the person for whom an LD is suspected. These tests are designed to detect cognitive skill levels, academics, speech, language assessments, psychological determination based on age, motor skills, and vocational potential.

Intellectual Disability

Intellectual disability refers to the condition in which an individual exhibits limited capacity for reasoning or functions at a lower intelligence level. Co-existing with this is the lack of ability in communication with others, limited skills in self-care, and limited social skills. Ability to function at a level allowing for successful employment can be obtained, however. Some experts recommend that rehabilitation counselors focus less on what the individual cannot do, but rather can do. Research has shown that dependent upon the level of intellectual disability, some individuals can be taught simple tasks which can lead to gainful steady employment and increased independence. With this attitude the counselor has an increased likelihood of finding suitable employment for the individual based on his or her strengths rather than weaknesses.

Causes of Intellectual Disability

The root cause of intellectual disability can be classified into two groups: genetic and physical. Genetically, the most common form is known as Down's Syndrome, which is the additional genetic material found on the 21st chromosome. A great risk is incurred if the mother is over age 35, as the child has a higher probability of developing Down's Syndrome. PKU is also a cause of intellectual disability. Testing in newborns is conducted to detect high levels of phenylalanine in the blood. If it is found, a phenylalanine-restrictive diet is maintained to limit the degree of intellectual disability. Tay-Sachs disease generally results in early mortality and is the result of metabolic disorder. Physical causes can include use of drugs, alcohol, tobacco, and environmental factors that can inhibit development of the fetus. Additionally maternal illness such as diabetes, toxoplasmosis, syphilis, or exposure to radiation, physical trauma either during pregnancy or delivery can lead to intellectual disability.

Psychiatric Disorders

An individual with a psychiatric disability suffers from a wide variety of emotions. These impairments make it challenging in maintaining employment. Oftentimes, the person initially sought help at the insistence of a family member or employer. The more severe the mental disorder, the less likely the person will have successful vocational potential. Emotions associated with these disorders can range from low motivation, fatigue, high stress levels, isolation, lethargy, catatonia, and anxiety. These are not traits that allow for a successful work environment. The counselor must determine if there is any potential for employment through a vocation profile, job analysis, and assessment of the individual's work motivation. Additionally, this type of disability could require lifelong reliance on medication, hospitalizations, outpatient treatment that could render stable employment a challenge.

Rehabilitation counselors can expect to see more clients with the most common disabilities. In the class of psychiatric disorders, these can involve disorders such as mood, anxiety, schizophrenia, sexual, sleep, eating, personality, dementia, and substance related disorders. Psychiatric disorders can affect a person's ability to fully function in society. These can affect socially, through relationships with family members and others, or occupationally, hindering ability to gain, hold, or keep employment. Society places a stigma on those individuals with psychiatric disorders, even going so far as to label a person negatively, referring to the person as "violent" or "crazy". With these attitudes, individuals with these disorders face greater challenges and biases in gaining and keeping employment.

Alcoholism

Etiology is defined as the study of causes and origins with roots based in the Greek language. There is not one single cause of alcoholism, yet there are many common factors. Genetically, children of an alcoholic parent have a greater likelihood of becoming alcoholics themselves, but some research also points to environmental factors. This, like many others, can be construed as a learned behavior. Some ethnic cultures such as Native American, Hispanic, Irish, and African-Americans, have traditionally had heavy usage of alcohol. As such, these groups have a higher dependency resulting in alcoholism. Additionally, family history of other drug abuse such as marijuana, tobacco, cocaine, can lead to tendencies towards alcohol addiction.

Alcoholism Disability

Most alcoholics began as social drinkers, often in their late teens. As the drink is introduced into the system a gradual tolerance builds up and it requires more levels of alcohol to gain the same effect. With this increase in tolerance, the body is accustomed to absorption of greater amounts of alcohol and in turn, the liver cannot process as well as it used to. The individual thus is well on his way to an addiction to alcohol. Dependence upon alcohol is defined as wanting to quit but not meeting with success, spending time in the acquisition of alcohol in social activities rather than spending time on work or familial responsibilities, and also in denying that there is an a problem to begin with. This disability is a disease, which if left untreated can lead to severe physical consequences and sometimes death.

Indicators of Alcohol Abuse

Regardless of whether an individual admits to possible alcohol use and addiction, there are several common physical and psychological factors that can provide a strong indicator to the counselor. These can include agitation, irritability, odor of alcohol present on person's breath or clothing, and flushed skin and red eyes, often leading to the individual wearing sunglasses even while indoors. The person may also exhibit depression, mood swings, anger, hostility and lashing-out at others, and even thoughts of suicide. Notably, the alcoholic has amassed skills in deceiving others to the extent of his addiction. It is often realized that this person is the last to accept the fact that he may have a problem. It is up to the counselor to assist the individual in realizing the extent of his problem and to guide him on the path to self-independence and the process of ending the addiction.

Drug Abuse

The primary goal of return to work from drug abuse includes the initial detoxification, counseling, developing a strong support system, and allowing for the return to a healthy, positive living environment. Building up the individual's self esteem is important as well since it can directly influence the individual's success in maintaining the goal of return to work. If the mindset is such that the person will not succeed, then chances are great that they will not. Vocational profiles are important in that an individual recovering from drug abuse may not have a steady work history from which to build on. In this case, you would then seek transferable skills to create a new career and work with other agencies experienced in placing individuals recovering from work in a suitable job situation. A structured environment is best in establishing positive drug free behaviors.

Disclosing Past Drug Abuse

Some insurance companies do not recognize drug abuse as a disability unless it was a direct result of an injury sustained on the job. Therefore, an individual with a history of drug abuse could be at a disadvantage in that disclosure of their disability could prohibit employment. This dilemma constitutes a barrier to employment and can lead to feelings of depression, lack of confidence, and lowered self-esteem. Fear of leaving the relative safety of a therapeutic environment and into the unknown territory of work can leave the individual with feelings of hopelessness and insecurity about the return to work as a whole. Counselors need to exhibit patience and understanding at this time and a willingness to assist with the process of return to work. While honesty is the best policy, deep thought and evaluation is required prior to disclosing past drug abuse on an application as hiding the problem may be seen as falsifying information on the application.

Withdrawal Symptoms

Drug abuse affects the central nervous system, blocking neural transmitters. As a result of withdrawal from the drug, one experiences negative physical and psychological symptoms. When withdrawal of the drug takes place, a person goes through a process known as detoxification. Without the drug, the body undergoes severe cravings for the drug and longs for the "high" produced by the drug. Stronger physical reactions to the withdrawal can include muscle spasm, twitching, seizures, coma, and even hallucinations or death. Psychologically, the person can experience frustration, depression, mood swings, and even suicidal tendencies. It is imperative that the rehabilitation counselor works closely with the treating physician in designing a disability management plan that considers any long lasting ill effects from the past drug use and also continuing education of the client to facilitate their reintroduction as a productive member of society.

Treatment of Drug Abuse

Three forms of treatment for drug abuse are as follows: outpatient methadone programs, residential stay programs, and at home treatments. Methadone treatments serve as a substitute for heroin and allow the medical team to focus on treating the individual socially and psychologically while allowing his body to gradually attain a drug-free state. A residential facility involves a stay of several weeks in which the individual undergoes communal counseling, management of withdrawal symptoms by the medical staff and gradual education of new drug-free coping mechanisms and increased self-esteem. This program also focuses on shared experiences with other individuals who have faced similar problems. At home treatment involved the individual enrolling in various programs within the community to assist with decreased drug dependence. Each method varies in the effectiveness and the rehabilitation professional should conduct a thorough assessment prior to recommending a particular method over another.

Employment Leaves and Benefits Administrations

Benefits and Outside Resources for Clients

There are many county, state, and national resources available that provide assistance in caring for your client. In the example of alcoholism, you have any number of chapters of 12 step programs located in many metropolitan areas. Additionally, the National Council on Disability provides a listing of state resources, assisted living resources, state mental health resources, and also a listing of vocational and rehabilitation agencies. There are also organizations and support groups which assist family members of those affected with a disability, such as Al-Anon. For the younger clients, there are agencies devoted to their care in many areas, including ensuring their right to an education. For permanently disabled clients, one needs to research additional federal aid such as Medicare and Social Security Disability insurance.

Legal Compliance in Disability Management

Under the Americans with Disability Act of 1990, no individual with a defined disability shall be denied the right to seek employment, nor be denied employment as a result of their disability. Companies can expect to make reasonable accommodations that do not cause an undue hardship on themselves in meeting the needs of their disabled employees whether it be in physical accommodations, providing assistance in terms of a reader, sign interpreter, or equipment modification to meet those needs. Utilizing the company legal department, medical consultations, as well as outside agency resources to provide the best possible work environment will ensure that all areas have been met with compliance.

Employees Health Benefits

In the workplace, an employer has some degree of influence over the health and welfare of their employees. Providing a safe working environment through safety training and prevention is a top priority. However, the individual has some responsibility in maintaining a healthy lifestyle too. Smoking, alcohol abuse and drug abuse do nothing to help the body and can often lead to a worksite accident if the person is under the influence. As a method of promoting a healthy lifestyle, companies are offering benefits such as onsite fitness facilities, access to nutritionists and dietitians, and a host of wellness programs. Additionally, making ergonomic changes to each workstation and other methods to the feet, hands, knees, and backs will minimize the possibility of a debilitating injury or accident. Making these changes results in cost savings over time.

Program Development, Management, and Evaluation

Benefits of a Disability Management Program

In a disability management program, the focus is on creating an ideal scenario in which to encourage a person to return to work. Working with an employer, the rehabilitation counselor can help the employer achieve greater worker health and productivity, employee retention through ongoing accommodation of the needs of the disabled person, safety and awareness, and increased business intelligence due to retaining talented employees. Short-term expenditures in disability management will yield great cost returns over the long haul. It is imperative that appropriate disability management programs are in place to ensure that the United States remains at the forefront of our global economy. Also, companies cannot afford to lose well-trained employees to remain competitive. Finally, there is more of a cost savings in keeping a disabled person employed versus paying out disability benefits.

Components of a Disability Management Program

Initially a needs assessment must be completed to evaluate the situation that led to the disability. A committee is thus formed to coordinate the facilitation of the plan. The committee establishes policies and procedures. A case manager who has relationships built with supporting community agencies is appointed. Employment opportunities would be identified that offer flexibility in work for a disabled person. The people within a company who are most likely to be involved in a disability situation are provided with the proper training. Additionally procedures dealing with data collection and evaluation are put into place. Finally, prevention strategies are outlines and appropriate expenditures are made to encourage greater safety awareness and accident prevention. With this comprehensive plan, a company can be better prepared to head off any potential problems in the event of an individual developing a disability on the job.

Needs Assessment

In a needs assessment, the rehabilitation counselor looks for information to classify as a baseline in determining the ideal management plan for a disabled person. It can include information such as the makeup of the workforce. This includes a statistical count of employees in terms of gender, age, ethnic backgrounds, and level of education attained. Analyzing this data can help an organization perfect the potential need for disability services and can highlight which groups may be affected. A history of disability in the workplace is important because it can measure the likelihood of injuries by department as well as forming a baseline in which improvements can be measured. A needs assessment can also provide an outline of common organizations and agencies that provide care and services to those affected by a disability. Finally, by evaluating past experiences of those who have already worked with and employed people with disabilities one can gain a greater understanding of practices that had a positive outcome versus those which did not.

Data Collection

In order to determine the degree to which a plan is meeting the needs of the people it's designed to help: a disabled individual, the informative collection of data must be completed at every step in the process. Methods for collecting this information involve determining what has already taken place in the attempt to meet the needs of the disabled person. Collection of this information is only useful so far as the analysis of the data is completed. This data may be collected by various employees at a company with the intent of sharing it between departments. This is not as much of an issue at a smaller company where you may find one individual serving multiple roles. The data may be in the form of monitoring attendance records or production numbers, monitoring in dollars the amount of money spent on a person's disability from the employer's perspective, etc. Without this data, there are no ways of benchmarking improvements to the policy and to make future recommendations.

Data Collection Process

In evaluating the success of a disability management program, it is imperative that data collection is performed on all areas of the program and from all active professional staff members. This can include notes that were taken on behalf of the coordinating committee, case managers, supervisors, and any community resources. Any minutes from meetings, log books, and activity reports should also be evaluated. If any special reports were conducted, such as monthly status reports on an individual's progress, this should also be included. Additionally, the regular reports used by Worker's Compensation, Employee Assistance Program, benefits, risk management, or other departments must be included in the data evaluation of the program.

Cost-Benefit Evaluation

While research has shown that companies are increasing their awareness of case management, initial findings show that it is cost effective to implement a case management program in terms of savings over the reduction in medical costs and disability payouts. Finding this information can be tricky, however, but it begins with collecting data on the individuals who are in the process of receiving treatment for disabilities or who have already begun receiving monetary benefits as a result of the disability. Tracking the demographics of the individuals, types of disabilities, and length of time out of work can be calculated, as can the absenteeism and retention rates of those employees who do return to the work force. Long term and short term data collection provides an on-going objective manner in which to determine the success of the program in terms of cost.

Monitoring and Evaluating

In order to properly evaluate the disability management system, data must be collected in regards to the types of injuries sustained, departments in which the injuries occurred, and also duration of the injury just to name a few. This data may also be collected to evaluate costs of the system to see if there are savings incurred with close management of a person's disability. It is imperative also to monitor the system to see how people are referred it, how assessments are handled, and also specifics on the intervention process. Additionally, ways in which the case manager closes each particular file and also whether or not injuries received any follow-ups would also be specifics to monitor and evaluate the success of the program and offer ways to make improvements.

Continuity of the Disability Management Plan

With as much preparation that goes into developing the disability management plan, a company should plan for the method to sustain its commitment to the goals of the program long after the initial excitement has worn off. Continued evaluation of the disability management program and policy changes as needs arise should be done on an on-going basis. This will ensure that through monitoring, no aspect of the program will lag behind. Monitoring of the effect on production, morale, and job satisfaction should be included in the data. Staff training could be encouraged and can include newly hired employees. Training team members in accident prevention and making them aware of behaviors that can contribute to a disabling condition increases their knowledge of disability management. Finally, through networking of the internal staff and outside organizations, the company gains the reputation as one focusing on prevention and disability management.

Data Analysis

Simply put, the amount of data that can be collected to evaluate the disability management program is enormous considering the large numbers of people involved in a disabled person's care. Organizing the questions into distinct categories can help in sorting through the information and evaluating its effectiveness. First, how well did the program meet the needs of the people it was designed to help? Second, did the operational aspects of the program perform their job thoroughly? Finally, were the program goals met and was policy followed through on every step of the process? By examining the data and answering these questions, can one get a sense of the effectiveness of the program and can make any future recommendations which could improve the program for future participants.

Disability Program Operations Evaluation

In defining the success of the disability management program operations aspects, questions such as whether the referrals to the program were made in a timely fashion. Additionally, determining whether there was good communication and smooth functioning of all departments in terms of reports and data being shared. The knowledge that all departments were functioning well and on the same page, so to speak is important to the evaluation. The case managers must also be aware of who is completing the program and who is not. The information must be gathered on those not completing the program to determine why he or she did not return to work or who did not perform well once back on the job.

Monitor Program

In evaluating the care of an individual, it is important to note whether the client felt as if the program was responsive and met his or her needs. Questions to be asked during the evaluation could include topics such as whether a person was quickly referred into the program, whether emotional issues were responded to by case manager referrals to community agencies, or also whether or not the case manager or other program workers were available and provided the right amount of assistance necessary. The idea being that the program was not a success unless the main participant, the disabled individual, was satisfied with the program.

Follow-Up Survey

Evaluating the program ensures that any problems are addressed immediately and also determining, from the client's perspective, how well the program addressed his or her needs. The case manager should allow sufficient time from ending the program to completion of the survey to allow the client time to readjust to the work environment. The types of questions to be included should cover whether the person was able to remain at work weeks, or even months, later. It also should ask what types of accommodations were made and if they were still necessary. Also, if any new problems arose as a result of the disability, perhaps if it has recurred. Finally, the case manager should be rated on his or her performance in meeting the needs of the individual. These ratings would determine if there are any changes that need to be made to the disability management program.

Preparing an Analysis

There are several software packages available specific to social work that can tabulate the information to answer virtually any question that one can devise. Common software packages can include the Statistical Package for the Social Sciences (SPSS) or the Statistical Analysis System (SAS). Other packages are available, but these two are specifically designed to deal with the compiling the data as it relates to the industry. Once the software package has been identified and the data entered, then the criteria must be set that needs to be processed. Benchmarking data should be set from which all other data can be measured. Past performance versus present performance could be statistically analyzed. Also, the predictor of future behavior could be measured out using trends from past data.

Depending on the audience, it is important to present the final analysis in a way in which the average person could read the data and understand the information it contains. A case manager may need the information separated by case, however, the case manager's supervisor may need the information presented to encompass all the cases the manager has worked on in the last quarter, for example. A coordinating committee may need an even broader encompassing view of the cases completed at one facility. It is important to understand the audience reading the report as well as tailoring the information specific to the needs of that person. Other departmental information that is not pertinent should not be included. Determining also the duration and frequency of the reporting is of great concern. Each reporting period offers the opportunity for additional opportunities to correct flaws in the system and produce better results the next time.

Success Rate

The effectiveness of a case management program can be measured in how well the employer adheres to the following: management team supporting the case management program, maintaining open lines of communication between service providers and the employee and case manager, and identifying benchmarks and other measuring tools to track progress of the plan. Additionally, the ability to maintain flexibility of the disability management plan and making changes to the policy as needed contribute to the success of the program. The success of the disability management plan can also be due to the similarity between the company's philosophical and ethical mission statements to the ideals stated within the disability plan.

In determining the success of the program, one must ask whether any preventative methods have been practiced in the workplace and whether they resulted in fewer injuries on the job. Also, deciding if the number of workers out on either long or short-term disability has been reduced due to these measures. It is a good idea to measure the intangible aspects such as the morale and job satisfaction of those individuals who have returned to work as well as those of his or her co-workers. Most importantly, the cost factors and any medical savings should be measured as well as the reduction in the number of claims for either Worker's Compensation or disability benefits payments.

Internal Case Management Program

When a company retains control of a disability case management program, they have greater power over the policy-making and can thus shape the program to fit within the company mission and philosophy. The program can be customized to the employer and allows for quick responses between departments. Communication is enhanced and work accommodations are easily facilitated as the caseworker most likely has familiarity and knowledge of the individual's job description and can make changes to allow the worker to continue in his or her old position in a more efficient manner. An internal case management program also identifies the company's commitment to fostering a partnership between the company and the employee. Planning and implementation can involve all levels of staff members from top management down in creating the internal plan.

Outsourcing a Case Management Program

A company has the right to choose a case manager who may be employed from within the company or through an external vendor. Internally, the person selected to be case manager may be assigned to either the human resources, medical, or benefits departments. Externally, an insurance company, social services, or a rehabilitation or vocational facility may employ the case manager. The choice may be made within a smaller company to outsource the case management to a company that has more experience and can bring to the table case scenarios that a smaller company may not have dealt with. A larger company, on the other hand, may want to have more control over disability case management and can distribute accordingly the administrative tasks involved in case management among a larger staff.

Selecting a Case Management Program Vendor

In selecting an external case management program vendor, there is a set of criteria that allows a comprehensive "apples to apples" comparison between vendors who've applied for contracts within a company. The application process should include the same set of questions asked of all potential vendors. Detailing areas of specialization and the educational background of the staff members, plus a listing of all services offered and supported by the vendor would enlighten the company as to the types of services to be expected. Also, detailing the fee schedule and what is included in each charge is important. These charges could be negotiated. The size of the case manager's workload and what amount of time the company can expect to be devoted to them can be included. Privacy policies and liability insurance should be provided for review. Most importantly, any references from other organizations that have contracted with a particular vendor may prove to be invaluable.

External Case Management Vendor Benefits

A smaller company is more likely to choose an external case management program because the ability of the external vendor to bring resources and past experience is greater than any the company could achieve on it's own. The program already has been tested and proven within other companies the vendor may be able to provide any suggestions to the program that the company may not have thought out. Additionally, having the external vendor as the authority and mediator in case management relieves the company from any potential conflicts or disputes between the employee and the company. Having few disability cases at a worksite may also be a reason to hire an external vendor so that the company would not have to pay a person to perform the case management duties on a full basis. Overall, cost is a consideration since having an experienced vendor in case management can reduce the learning curve and therefore time spent in managing a disability case and return to work scenario.

Barriers to the Development of a Comprehensive Disability Management Plan

Promoting an effective comprehensive disability management plan is an uphill battle because a company can encounter many obstacles to their goal. Promoting a plan of safety awareness and healthy lifestyles needs to receive "buy-in" from some of the key players in a company. The best method of achieving this is through the management team at all levels but in particular from the top down. If the supervisors believe in the benefits of the disability management plan, then they are more likely to encourage a disabled individual to remain at work. Additionally, the supervisor does not lose the skill set of a worker and thus, forced to train a new employee; rather they can retain a talented worker with minimal disruption.

Challenges in Disability Management

The majority of organizations are resistant to change. Although an organization is considered an entity as a whole, it is comprised of many individuals, each of whom has individualized thoughts, opinions, and ideas as to how the organization should be run. Getting this group to buy in and support disability management as a whole can be challenging. The hierarchy and structure of a company is well set and generally in the form of organizational chart, however, influences from others can also play a role in how well received a new initiative can be. One influence on the decision-making and acceptance of a disability management plan may be the size of the organization. Larger groups can rely on more personnel to meet these new tasks whereas a smaller company may have to increase hiring or assign additional tasks to key members. A second influence can be cost, again, where a larger company may be more readily able to absorb additional costs in meeting accommodations, but a smaller one may not.

Responsibilities a Coordinating Committee

A coordinating committee is made up of all the departments who are actively involved in meeting the needs of a disabled individual in the workforce. These can include the management team, human resources, benefits department, safety team, training, Employee Assistance Program (EAP), production, risk management, and legal. Working together to ensure the best work environment via accommodations, the focus of the coordinating committee is on developing administrative procedures to follow when a need for services is brought to the attention of the employer, ensuring that each member of the team is aware of any problems with the disabled individual in the workforce as well as reviewing of cases and how progress is made for the individual. This committee also has the authority to determine if any changes need to be made to the policy based on a disabled person's experience. Additionally, the committee can serve as an advocate for the disabled individual to any outside agencies.

EAP

An Employee Assistance Program is designed to assist all employees and their families through confidential services provided for any substance, mental or physical condition as it affects their job. The majority of the people who consult EAP, however, seek help with substance abuse or emotional problems. This leaves a great number of people without access to services in which the EAP already has formed contacts with throughout the community. Research has shown that through their experience and potential to help a disabled individual, more awareness needs to be made to focus on referring those individuals to the EAP. Staff members who work under the EAP umbrella generally have more experience than other departments such as benefits or risk management in handling these cases, however, the EAP has not been fully utilized for disability management.

Training Key Personnel

As the disability management plan takes shape, key roles are assigned to various staff members in the workplace. These employees need to be trained properly to ensure that their role is thoroughly understood in the overall scheme of the plan. Additionally, they need to be made aware of the procedures for their particular role. For example, a front line manager of a person who has been injured on the job needs to be observant of the issues that can arise from lack of early intervention and be aware of meeting those needs head on. All members with the potential to be directly involved in a disability management scenario would also need an understanding of the policy as a whole. For those staff members taking on additional responsibilities in other areas, such as safety or risk management, will also need training in those fields.

Training Staff Members

Training of not only the key players in disability management, but also in all staff members creates a company environment in which a disabled person has the same opportunities as all the other employees. This training allows all members to perpetuate the belief that disability management is something to be expected and common in the workforce, rather than rare and hard to obtain. In the training, the staff members are taught that disability management tasks should be part of the everyday work environment and shown how each job function can be amended to include these disability management tasks. In designing the training, it should be decided who needs the training, who will perform the training, what would be the content, and the duration of the training. Additionally, determining which jobs are best suited for the front lines of disability management should be identified.

Workplace Intervention for Disability Prevention

Disability Management

Disability management not only covers how to involve a disabled person in a return to work scenario, but also in preventing work related disabilities in the first place. The concept of disability management involves using a person's skills and abilities to best minimize the effect on the employer in terms of cost and also to encourage a worker to return to work as quickly as possible for increased self-esteem and satisfaction. With this in mind, a company can expect to see higher profitability, increased employee productivity, and greater employee retention. Additionally, a company can expect to see a decrease in the disability disbursements, absenteeism will be on the decline, employee morale and loyalty will be on the rise. It is important to note also that compliance with the ADA and other legislation will be achieved.

Prevention

While a good disability management plan is essential to create an ideal working environment for a person who has been injured on the job, the preferred goal that most companies would like to meet is that of being accident free. Accomplishing this takes dedication on behalf of the employer in creating the safest work environment possible for their employees. Teaching one's staff to avoid injuries and illness can help reduce costs and ensure that the work environment is safe for all employees, regardless of prior disability status. Along with safety training and thorough job training for each skill, companies must follow guidelines set by federal standards and OSHA for the industry. Some industries have higher OSHA guidelines based on the nature of their business. Information collected on those accidents resulting in injury or disability must be evaluated and proper correctional changes made to reduce the risk in the future.

Prevention in Disability Management

Preventing an accident in the workplace is more cost-effective than managing the care of one who is injured at work. Prevention programs are developed to help reduce the number of accidents or injuries at work, but also to show the workers that the employer is dedicated to the well-being of their employees and also on their morale and satisfaction. In designing these prevention programs, the employer should look to the ways in which each worker performs his or her job. In this manner, they can customize their prevention strategy on each specific job. For example, designating lower lifting requirements may help reduce the number of back injuries, or instead of lifting, creating an automated assembly line. The employers can also insure that any changes made fall in line with cost-cutting measures while maximizing employee safety.

Prevention Measures

Based on the data analysis, a company may discover that ergonomics plays a large role in the prevention of workplace injury. Changing table heights or chair heights could lead to few back injuries among workers who primarily sit on the job. The data may show a need to increase the use of safety equipment such as using hard hats in high-risk areas, or protective eyewear and earpieces. Some prevention methods may require additional training in best practices for a task such as lifting. An educational program may be initiated that focuses on diet and nutrition to reduce the risks associated with lack of exercise and a poor diet. A company may decide to create a health care or wellness facility onsite to be used by all employees.

Preventative Measures

Through the compliance with OSHA regulations and installing preventative programs at work aimed at decreasing the number of accidents and injuries, a company can see their costs of disabilities go down. Investing in wellness programs and educating staff members on the benefits of healthy lifestyles can also decrease the incidences of injury at the worksite. Proper job training and safety measures have cut down on the numbers of accidents as more responsibility is given to the employee to ensure that procedures are being followed. With the addition of automated manufacturing processes, the risk of injury has also declined as more of the work is being done by machine versus a person. With a company culture focused on preventative measures, the employer can see dramatic costs decreases to the disability benefits payouts.

Ergonomics

Ergonomics is defined as the method of maximizing worker productivity but not at the expense of worker fatigue, physical pain, or discomfort. It has special importance for a disabled individual considering modifications may need to be made in the work environment as well as company building in order to comply with creating a suitable work area to accommodate the disability. Some common job modifications may be adjustments to equipment such as an ergonomic chair, height adjustments on a desk, phone adjustments, lighting adjustments, larger computer screen, or an ergonomic keyboard. Without taking ergonomics into account, a company can run the risk of potential future health problems or injuries that can incur higher medical costs and potential litigation. For the amount of money that a company may spend on these small changes, there is a greater benefit and yields higher returns in the form of productivity and employee morale.

Change Agent

In making any organizational change, it is often one person who can clearly identify the need to make changes that benefit the organization as a whole. A change agent is the crux in beginning the process to make a change. The person in this position usually does not gain any public recognition and also may work alone. The best person suited for this position is one who is thorough in their research and able to speak with all levels of management and to seek out those who can be influential in decision-making. Identifying the key players and focusing on the goal will enable the change agent to make new processes and procedures occur in the workplace.

Policy

Policy serves as the outline and structure system in which all processes and procedures are derived. In order to properly manage a method for preparation in dealing with an individual, a framework must be put in place in which all people can expect the same method of care under this plan. The rights of all disabled individuals versus others must be equal. Another aspect to a disability policy is that the benefits that relate to a disabled individual such as services, performance reviews, training, etc. are all brought together and are outlined to meet the needs of all disabled individuals. This provides the guidelines for future long-term plans. In addition, the disability management policy must be flexible in order to respond to individual issues and also able to respond to changes in the system. In order for an entire organization to support this plan, it must be reviewed by all levels of management and appear in written form accessible to everyone.

Policy Phase of Disability Management

A succinct policy involves identification of information that is relevant to a person who is disabled. The ideal information in a policy would include who is covered under the plan and detailing the criteria to make that judgment. Also, outlining the benefits that one can expect to receive under the policy must be included in a manner that is easy to comprehend. The timeline in which an individual can expect to see action once a debilitating injury has occurred should be included. Additionally, identification of how the policy will be implemented and that information will be communicated to the individual should be outlined. Providing information of the disability management system to all key players as well as employees is the main goal to accomplish.

Accomplish Objectives of a Policy

In relaying information about the corporate culture, an ideal stated and written policy would provide employees with the knowledge that the company values its employees and recognizes that they are valuable assets. Creating a positive environment to encourage disabled employees to return to work in the most efficient manner and return to productive roles cements the partnership that should ideally exist. Working together to offer solutions to creating a safe work environment resulting in increased morale and loyalty, rather than creating a negative hostile work environment has shown an effect on the rapidity in which a disabled employee recuperates faster.

Common Objectives

One common factor in creating a disability management plan is to decrease the costs associated with a disability plus keeping the individual in constant communication with the employer to encourage and facilitate a quicker return to work. The employer is able to spend less money on disability payments and worker's compensation and can focus on developing a health and wellness attitude and a safer work environment. Time lost by a disabled employee is decreased and the attitude of working in partnership with the employer versus against is encouraged. Fewer employers would seek outside legal counsel and job security would be heightened due to the understanding that the company does not want to lose highly trained and skilled employees.

Individual Objectives

Underscoring the need for buy-in of a disability management plan, each key player looks to find ways in which they will directly benefit if certain goals are met. In the example of a line supervisor, a goal may be to meet 100% of production. If one of the employees becomes disabled, their goal may be amended to meet 80% of production. Utilizing worksite accommodations, the supervisor can arrange to have the disabled worker return to work in a capacity while not at the original goal, can still help meet production needs. Both parties have thus benefited from this arrangement. Return to work can also help with a reduction in medical costs and therefore a reduction in cost to the employer. The supervisor can help his employee retain job skills and also can protect the individual's income.

Indication of Employer Support

In researching a company, several common denominators are found that indicate a company's responsiveness to disability management. A formal Employee Assistance Program (EAP) is in place and the company offers a comprehensive health insurance package indicated a strong believe in supporting employees. Also, company that spend minimal amounts on long term and short term disability plans for it's employees indicate that they value them and want to ensure that they are taken care of if an injury occurs. Companies who offer training programs and who are willing to make accommodations or make changes in the jobs themselves are open to communications and suggestions from other members of the team. This open policy indicates that they have either in the past had experience working with disabled employers or supports their efforts in the workplace.

Employer Responsiveness

For those employees who have received a disability at work, the way the company responds to their needs plays a direct role in how effective the disability management program could be. Employers who offer assistance in the form of prompt referrals to a case management program, or who maintain constant contact with the employees while out on leave generate more satisfied employees in the workforce due to their expressed concern. Additionally, the programs referred to by the case manager and also the concern from the case manager themselves lead the individual to feel as though the employer has a vested interest in his recovery. Keeping the lines of communication open both before and after an injury are imperative in responding to the individual's needs as the problems arise, thus minimizing any opportunities for dissatisfaction to occur.

Department's Role

In developing a program for disability management, the benefits department generally has the greatest amount of responsibility towards meeting those goals. Their role is to evaluate claims and provide compensation based on an investigation into the disability. They also serve to act as a mediator for outside agencies and if necessary, counsel employees throughout the transition in returning to work. The EAP provides support often in the form of referrals to outside agencies as in services for substance abuse addiction. They also can help the families of those suffering from the disability by providing confidential support services. The risk management department serves as the administrator of the worker's compensation plan and the legal department provides advice concerning the administration of the benefits and ensures that the company is in legal compliance with the ADA and EEOC.

Large Company Versus Smaller Company

Although cost cutting measures are important for all companies, it is more imperative at a smaller company who may not have the necessary resources to support the wellness and preventative programs that a larger company can. A large company can budget for an onsite wellness facility and exercise room, but a smaller company cannot. Money made be more readily available to fund these programs but a smaller company can also provide cost cutting measures through training on workplace safety and training. A larger company may have established channels of communication with both existing employees and new hires, whereas a smaller one may tend to create the policy as they go along. Finally, a larger company may have the capacity to employ a full time case manager and maintain a database of past worker's compensation claims, but a smaller company may direct the care to an outside agency instead.

Discriminatory Practices

Discrimination based on a disability is tantamount to violation of one's civil rights. The Equal Employment Opportunity Commission (EEOC) is responsible for enforcing non-discriminatory hiring practices and treatment of employees in the workforce. This can include practices in hiring, interviewing, and extension of a job offer, to distribution of work assignments, arranging work transfers, training in different aspects of the job, wages, and other practices including termination. The EEOC and the ADA ensure that workplace decisions are not based upon a company's perceptions of an individual's capabilities or limitations. Rather, the company is expected to coordinate an individual's job based on whether they can perform the essential duties of the position. This may include making reasonable accommodations to enable an individual to perform his or her job. If an employer does not choose to make these accommodations, then they can be discriminating against the individual.

Essential Function

Essential functions are defined as those duties crucial to an individual's job. What constitutes as essential for one position may not be for another. Based on the person's skills and the required tasks for the job, the amount of work required to perform the job is measured as a percentage. A higher percentage indicates a greater level of an "essential function" of that particular job. For example, a security guard may measure walking a facility as 80-90% of the job. A security supervisor may have walking as only 50% of the job with the remainder made up of administrative tasks performed at a desk. If a disabled individual cannot walk the required amount to be a security guard, then the job may be accommodated to include a greater amount of paperwork. Written job descriptions are invaluable to a disability management plan in that they define each job in specific terms of types of tasks to be performed, percentage of time each task should take and qualitative goals for the task in a given time period.

Undue Hardship

When researching accommodations for a person with a disability, an employer must look to the costs involved in meeting that accommodation. Under the Americans with Disabilities Act, it states that an employer is obligated to make reasonable accommodations for an employee as long as meeting that need does not pose an undue hardship to the employer. By "undue hardship", the Act means that which causes a burden in terms of cost in meeting the need, restructuring of the workflow is not possible, or making the accommodation would alter the nature of the business. In such instances, the Act states that failure to make the accommodation because of the above reasons is considered non-discriminatory. One such example of undue hardship is when a company finds that the only individual able to perform the duties of a job is no longer capable. If there is no suitable accommodation that would allow the person to perform the job, then the company has undue hardship in meeting that requirement.

Transferable Skills

Transferable skills are defined as those skills learned in a position requiring some degree of complex work activity. These skills may be taught on the job or through vocational or education training, but are not picked up in a matter of a few short days. These skills require specialized training to the employer or within the industry. Examples of transferable skills would be running a piece of machinery, programming said piece, using specific tools, using specialized equipment or measuring devices, etc. These skills require a learning curve of 30 days or more. Highly skilled work involves an individual's higher use of their judgment and understanding of a piece of machinery, concept, and relationship skills in dealing with other people to perform the daily aspects of the job. This level generally requires advanced education such as a degree or many more years of experience performing this type of work. The learning curve can be two years of greater at this level. Generally unskilled work, which is learned in 30 days or less and on the job, does not constitute transferable skills.

Four Groups for Vocational Purposes

1. Individuals who can return to their past work activities and job function
2. Individuals who should be retrained for another more suitable job

3. Individuals who are capable of working in a sheltered environment
4. Individuals who can only work under self-care

Sheltered or Home Environment

For some individuals, the idea of a return to work is not possible under the standard retraining scenario. Due to certain disabilities, a person needs a new environment in which to work and remain a productive member of the workforce. For instance, for a person who has COPD, environmental factors at work could exacerbate the condition. Dust, fumes, smoke, and excessive changes in temperature could affect one's breathing and cause additional lung problems, even with protective safety equipment. For these people, an environment in which specialized respiratory equipment such as an oxygen system is readily available will encourage a faster return to work and more likelihood to remain productive. Additionally, having the worksite at home can help to accommodate the lack of mobility and fatigue that can accompany certain disabilities will help the person live more independently.

Referral

In meeting the needs of a person injured on the job, the assigned case manager may first be made aware of an individual through application of worker's compensation or disability benefits. For a person who already has a disability, the supervisor who needs to make accommodations to the work area may consult the case manager. The benefits department may provide a list of people out on either short or long-term disability to the case manager. Identifying those people who are eligible for assistance through the disability management program should undergo training to recognize those people who are most likely to benefit. A specific process must be in place that recognizes the need for early intervention in getting these people the assistance they need.

Employer-Sponsored Benefits Verses Incidence of Worker's Compensation Claims

For those companies who have made a commitment to disability management through programs of early intervention, monitoring, and evaluation, the levels of disability related claims through Worker's Compensation have been on the decline. This can be partially accredited through the increase in preventative measures and safety training being performed at the worksite. Companies whose supervisors actively participate in workplace accommodations and reintroduction of workers immediately after return from time off for a disability generally report lower levels of claims overall. There is less likely to be ongoing accidents due to training and correction of procedures and the proper way to perform the job tasks to minimize injuries. Another aspect involves the degree to which the company culture supports an environment in which disability management and worksite safety takes a high priority.

Incentives for Supervisors and Managers

With the idea of retaining skilled and trained employees, a supervisor should look for ways to accommodate a disabled employee in the worksite. Understandably, under scrutiny to maintain production levels while working with a reduced staff, it is imperative to devise ways to meet both needs. Several companies are offering financial incentives for meeting the needs of disabled employees and reducing costs at the same time. For those supervisors who do not, the cost of disability payments may come out of their department budget. Holding a supervisor accountable for the number of accidents in his department would provide an incentive for him to create ways to make the workplace safer. Additionally, tailoring a portion of the performance appraisal on how well the supervisor accommodates a disabled individual is another incentive.

Costs

Employers generally tend to argue that the costs of accommodating a worker's disability are too high and therefore, cannot be met. This has been said in instances where an employer does not want to make the necessary adjustments to the work environment for one person. A case manager can inform the employer that compliance with the ADA and EEOC is mandatory and that research has shown that while accommodating a worker does not increase the bottom line, it does, however increase worker productivity. The loss in a skilled or trained worker remaining on disability does not occur and you increase the morale and financial state of an individual who may be anxious to return to work and improve his or her lot in life.

Managerial Attitude

In a research study, managers tended to find that those employees who returned to work were more likely to be more productive than workers who were not disabled. Additionally, the job performance was rated high on performance reviews, and the quality of work was the same or higher than that of non-disabled workers. Other measures include the additional willingness to work harder, better attendance records, and more punctuality on the job. Disabled workers were viewed as more reliable, possessed strong leadership characteristics, and had strong desires to be promoted to higher positions. Finally, managers reported that there was no difference in the manner in which they supervised disabled employees versus non-disabled. From their perspective, the benefits of disability management had paid for itself.

Employer's Perception of the Individual's Disability

A supervisor's attitude and flexibility plays a strong role in the length of time that an individual is out on disability leave. The number of weeks out on a disability is in direct proportion to the individual's belief of the likelihood of his or her return to work. Although the severity of a person's disability determines how long the recovery period will be, supervisors may occasionally put off the notion that a person would not be likely to return to work due to his or her preconceived notions of the recovery time. If this information is communicated to the individual, it may become a self-fulfilling prophecy that their recovery time will be much longer. Also, if there were any personality or performance issues between the employee and the supervisor, they may unknowingly pass those negative emotions onto the individual. Since the supervisor is a key player in accommodating the return to work for the individual, it may be necessary to ensure that the supervisor is accepting of the person's return to work and also in making sure all necessary accommodations are made.

Implementing a Disability Management Plan

Under the disability management plan, the employer needs to identify the specific information needed to outline the steps in the plan. For example, the policy should state when initial contact will be made and who will make the call to the employee who has been newly disabled. Also, identifying how long an employee's job will be held for his return and developing a list of expected accommodations needed upon his return should also be stated. By contacting various outside sources such as physicians, therapists, and other health care workers, in addition to line supervisors and managers will set the scene for open lines of communication between the employee and the employer. Establishing a data collection system to document progress and problems or issues as they arise is also necessary for management of the disability.

Newly Disabled Employee Eligibility

Once an injury has occurred on a job site, the employer then determines who would be a candidate for the disability management program. For some injuries, recovery time is minimal and can occur in a matter of days. A sprained ankle is one scenario and little to no intervention on behalf of the employer is needed. For other injuries that are more debilitating, the idea is on early intervention as a method to reduce costs, minimize lost time from work, and encourage a faster return to work. In these cases, identifying who falls in what category can be confusing. Employers are faced with the dilemma in determining who is eligible for disability management. Contacting all injured employees without regard to severity of injury can result in increased workload for those key players. However, only contacting those with certain injuries may exclude those who would benefit from the program. The company would need to determine set criteria to see who would best benefit using methods such as physician recommendations, duration of time off from work, or diagnosis of the injury.

Eligibility Criteria

The policy of disability management must outline additional guidelines for those qualified to receive care under the plan. This can include criteria for which individuals may qualify for physical therapy rather than simply rest at home. A determination could also be made in which employees recuperate at home and achieve a specified level of recovery prior to returning to work in even a part time capacity. A reduction in work hours may be necessary for an employee versus a return to full time work. Finally, determining the requirements for changing a person's job responsibilities versus keeping the individual at a lesser skilled position during the recovery period. Some companies choose to retire an employee who may have little to no chance of returning as a productive worker because of their disability and criteria must be identified in that scenario as well.

Disability Management Program Admission

In reviewing those employees who may benefit from the program, the case managers must be cautious in not automatically admitting everyone who is injured on the job, but rather, systematically select those individuals who are most likely to benefit. The criteria could be in the timeframe in which an individual has suffered from a disability. In other words, only selecting those individuals who have been out of work, say for 3 weeks or more. Or, selecting those individuals who have an existing disability prior to employment who are now finding it difficult to perform some aspects of his or her position. Also, if there is an employee returning to work after a non-work related injury, this person may need assistance in the process of returning to his duties at the old job.

Basic Intervention Categories

During the process of determining the interventions needed, the case manager should explore whether disclosure of the disability would help or hinder the return to work process and whether assistance is needed to negotiate any accommodations to be made to the work environment. At times, the supervisors and immediate co-workers may not understand the extent of a person's lack of ability to perform the job and may react in a negative manner. To alleviate this, it is sometimes necessary to inform them, while at the same time, not disclosing personal information about the individual. Here is one example where training and education of the workforce in general may come in handy with regards to a person's disability. Also, a review of the workplace policies regarding disability may need to be performed by the employer. The individual also needs to be aware of his or her legal rights in the event of negative feedback and attitudes regarding his work performance or his disability.

Documentation Process

Once a client has been identified as needing additional resources to implement his or her care, the case manager is responsible for tracking the information on a checklist. The list should include the workplace interventions, interventions with health care professionals and with social agencies. The case manager should also monitor the performance of these outside agencies to ensure that the best interests of the individual are being served. The intervention should note the type of action taken, date the action was taken, the outcome, and any follow-ups. Additionally, it should include in detail the actions taken such as additional education, job retraining, or physical changes made to the workstation. In keeping with the confidentiality policy, the intervention checklist should only include an ID number as the identifier of the individual.

Complete the Documentation

Once it becomes clear that the services provided by the disability management program are no longer needed, it becomes necessary to complete the documentation to close a case. A case may close due to a person recovering from his or her disability or when a worker's compensation situation ends when the person returns to work. In closing the case, the documentation needed should include whether or not the individual was able to return to work and in what capacity, whether it is a new job, new responsibilities, or whether the person did not return to work at all. Additionally, the documentation should include if the worker received any assistance from other services, through accommodations at work, or whether the person was assigned a new permanent position. Finally, a cost overview that includes amount of disability payments made, costs of medical benefits, and other expenses should also be included.

Eligibility to Teach

In order to provide the experience necessary to train new staff members on disability management, the company should look to top management initially to promote the concept to the team as a whole. This way they can cement their commitment to providing disabled individuals with a better work environment that would accommodate his or her limitations or restrictions. While top management can provide an overview of why a disability management plan would benefit the organization, they may need to bring in outside consultants or specialists who can provide more detailed expertise to the various departments that may be involved in managing this plan. Generally, these consultants would be brought in from departments of social work or rehabilitation facilities.

Training Session Content

In assisting with the disability management promotion, the supervisor is charged with the success of the program as a whole. His or her role is to identify those workers who will benefit from the program through assessments based on the person's ability to perform their job. This assessment can be based on how well the person meet's job goals, his or her attendance record, and any onsite accidents or injuries. The supervisor also would need to participate in any return to work program on behalf of the employee and also designate any accommodations that need to be made to accomplish this. The supervisor is also responsible for educating members of the department on the disability and the need to make changes for this person to perform his job. Finally, the supervisor is consigned to monitor the performance of this individual to determine if there is a need to make changes once the accommodations have been completed, or if there is a worsening of the disability.

Counteract the Resistance to Training

Any indication of a change in responsibilities and tasks can sometimes result in negative attitudes and unwillingness to meet this new challenge. While top management may support the creation of a disability management program, mid-level management or line employees may not buy into the system. When this occurs, the ones implementing these changes must look to the reasons why there is resistance and counteract those. Employees may feel that adding these tasks may already increase his or her workload. Management can ease this by removing other tasks or assigning these new tasks to workers whose schedules may not be as full. Additionally, the managers must set up a process for ongoing dialogue and support during this transition. Finally, to increase support of the disability management program, an incentive plan could be introduced to all those who will be adding these new tasks to the workload.

Inform Employees

Communication is an integral part of the disability management program. For current employees, it's imperative that they are aware of the services available to them in the event of a disability. Until the company has sustained this program for some time, it is their responsibility to ensure that all employees are aware of its existence through newsletters, posters on site, meetings, or from direct supervisors and management. For a new hire to the company, the management team or human resources should provide a description of the company culture and the program to enforce the philosophy that the company cares about its employee's well-being and safety. This information should be written in language that is easy to understand and in a format such as a brochure or posted on the company website.

Accommodations for a Disabled Client

To meet the needs of both the employer and employee in designing a suitable work environment, one must consider all factors such as physical limitation, needs for additional resources or equipment and also non-tangible job modifications. Physical changes can include height restrictions on a desk, chair or workstation, physical location of an office as it relates to less travel or walking from parking lot, restroom facilities, break rooms, or proximity to main entrance. Physical changes can also be made to the minimum job requirements in a warehouse environment with less heavy lifting, for example. Additional resources or equipment may involve hearing devices on telephones, headsets, speakerphones, larger computer monitors, voice activated software packages, assistants, sign language interpreters, or note takers. Modification of the job involves adjusting work hour start and end times, more sedentary work versus field work, and switching from full time to part time work with an adjusted salary.

Communication with the Disabled Person

In order to provide the individual with the ideal environment to return to work, it is imperative that open communication is done with the individual at the earliest moment possible. This is done to ensure that any accommodations that are needed can be researched and implemented. The thinking is that the person with the disability may have had the disability for some time and therefore be aware of the accommodations needing to be made. If the disability is a new one, then the individual will be the best at deciding what accommodations he or she will be able to work with. Additionally, some adaptations thought common to people with similar disabilities may not be the correct choice as no two people are alike, therefore, no two disabilities should be treated in the same manner. The best person to involve in determining the proper accommodations would be the person with the disability.

Resources

While communication is necessary with the individual and his or her supervisor on the need for adjustments to the workspace, other resources can be used to determine the likely changes to be made based on the type of disability the individual faces. The Job Accommodation Network (JAN) is a database listing over 4000+ accommodations that were made in the workforce and provides statistical analysis of how well these have worked. It provides a great amount of detailed information to assist companies, large and small, in meeting the needs of the disabled individuals in their workforce. The service is an excellent way for a case manager to present options to both the supervisor and the employee on ways to make the workspace more functional for the individual.

Rheumatoid Arthritis

Depending on the severity of the disease, the disabled individual may have limited functionality of the hands and feet and the person may experience swelling and stiffness in the joint first thing in the morning. One accommodation may be to alter the starting work time to allow the person greater mobility once some of the stiffness has passed. Changing from a job that requires a great deal of movement to one more sedentary will help since the person may experience difficulties in walking and moves more slowly. As the disease progresses, the person may have further limitations in range of motion and the hands may lose the ability to grasp, pinch, or pull. Accommodations to the workspace involving chair heights, closer parking spaces due to fatigue, and switching from medium to light work can aid the person with rheumatoid arthritis remain a functioning member of the company.

Work-Related Back Injury Limitations

Due to advanced age and a more sedentary lifestyle, our bodies do not have the abilities to take repeated wear and tear and still be as resilient as before. A physician may recommend physical therapy or surgery to correct any injuries to the back. For the employer, this means that an individual will need to have time constraints on his or her work time to allow for time off for appointments and the surgery itself. Once the individual returns to work, a lighter workload may be ordered as well as limitations placed on standing, stooping, lifting, or bending. The duration of the restrictions may be temporary in nature or permanent depending on how severe the injury was. In that case, the employer may need to consider permanent job changes for this person and possible retraining in other areas.

Back and Neck Pain

With the longevity of today's society, people can expect to have more "wear and tear" on their bodies as opposed to centuries ago. Unless people take care of their bodies, the deterioration can occur much faster. Overuse injuries at the worksite are very common. Two of the most common injuries occur in the back and the neck for several reasons. Lifting improperly, poor posture, poor nutrition to the body, little or no workspace ergonomics, and a more sedentary lifestyle can contribute to these injuries. Safety training is a must for any company and more so for those that require physical activity on the job. Along with the proper use of safety equipment, such as back supports, comes a decrease in the incidence of injuries on the job. As people age, the vices of years past come back in the form of less resilience and bounce back from certain injuries. Through education and awareness, companies can help to change this.

Male Individual, Age 22, with a T-12 SCI Vocational Rehabilitation Plan

With the average age of SCI patients as 31.5 years, the likelihood for vocational rehabilitation is greater than that of a person who is injured during middle age. The level of a T-12 injury is one where loss of function is at the lower thoracic region and just above the lumbar region. This allows for use of the mid to upper abdominals, upper chest and arms, and the neck area. Greater mobility is possible through the use of the arms to propel a wheelchair. A younger individual is more likely to have a higher employment rate due to ability to return to school and is more open to retraining. At the age of 22, this individual may have completed college and can utilize the degree in an administrative role. If the person has only completed high school, a career assessment would be in line to determine the person's interests and skills and then apply them to an environment capable of accommodating the disability.

Diabetes Job Counseling

There is little need for vocational rehabilitation for a person who keeps his diabetes well managed and under control. Usually a rehabilitation counselor is called upon to assist someone who already has developed complications from this disease. Utilizing a vocational profile, job analysis, and assessment of the individual, one can determine the extent of the disability and can create a plan suited for return to work. With diabetes, good management of insulin levels is key and scheduling the work environment to allow for insulin administration (if necessary), regular breaks and meals, and a consistent schedule rather than varying shifts allow the individual to control and manage their disability. Additionally, vision problems may need to be addressed with the employer and reasonable accommodations made to assist with the reduction in sight. Complications from amputation or neuropathy will need to be addressed to design a workspace allowing for the decrease in mobility and increase the level of comfort. Insulin levels can arise in stressful environments and changes to the work schedule or job responsibilities may need to be addressed to help the individual find a suitable work environment.

Accommodations for Production Line Worker with Severe Asthma

In following the guidelines as set by the ADA, the employer must make any accommodations that do not cause any undue hardship on the employer in order to provide a work environment adaptive to his disease. A workplace assessment will identify any triggers to stimulating an asthma attack. It is a given that the individual is following his medical treatment plan as outlined by his physician. At the worksite, such triggers may include pollutants, dust, or changes in temperature. In his job at the assembly line, the employer may insure that he has the proper safety equipment such as a dust mask or one that specially filters out minute particles. Also, if he is able to perform other duties such as paperwork processing, rather than assembly, it would be a reasonable request to do so. If stamina is an issue, use of a chair or additional break periods away from the assembly station can be enforced.

Prosthetic Limb Workplace Issues

Aside from the accommodations to be made for a person with a prosthetic limb, other devices may be used to make the job easier to perform. For a person with a double amputation of the lower extremities, use of a backpack to carry items from one location to another leaves the hands free to propel the chair. Also, tables that are set on wheels, other motorized carts, or scooters are useful. Tools that allow for longer reaches can benefit people with both lower and upper extremities amputated. The emotional aspect of the amputation should also be taken into account. Educating the person's department and supervisor on the limitations of the person as well as his or her strengths.

Multiple Sclerosis Barriers to Employment

Multiple sclerosis affects the body in many areas. Unfortunately, this results in many differing symptoms to occur that can be unpredictable and can render the person unable to perform the required duties of the position. Sensitivity to heat, causing increases in symptom occurrence in MS can be contained by providing an air-conditioned workspace and keeping the area much cooler. Periods of fatigue also occur which frequently is the cause for keeping an individual from gainful employment. The two MS related types of fatigue are muscle fatigue and idiopathic lassitude, which is overwhelming tiredness, not alleviated by rest. Problems with cognitive thinking are also related to MS since the majority of patients experience decreased attention spans and concentration, short term memory and impaired ability to use problem solving skills and reasoning. Finally, physical symptoms that can affect the ability to work include lack of motor skills, reduction in eyesight, chronic pain, and lack of coordination.

Epilepsy in the Work Environment

Overcoming any stigmas associated with the disease would be the primary concern for the rehabilitation counselor. An epileptic individual faces fear and apprehension due to the uncertainty of the disease. Coupled with the reactions normally encountered by others upon seeing a seizure in progress leads to feelings of embarrassment. In the work environment, consideration must be made to ensure the safety of the individual as well as those of the coworkers. Disclosure is an option for the individual; however, employers are required by the ADA to make the necessary accommodations for all people with a disability. Points to make with an employer could include information that attendance rates for a person with epilepsy are higher than those without, accident rates for non-epileptic individuals are higher, job site modifications can be easily made, and finally, that industrial insurance rates usually do not decrease upon hiring a person with epilepsy.

Rehabilitation Potential of a Person with a Learning Disability

As with any disability, the severity can affect the ability to successfully complete rehabilitation and come away with the skills necessary to function as an independent person. Ability to maintain control over the learning disability has been shown to have a profound effect on the success rate of an individual in all facets of life from employment, to independent living, to self-sufficiency. Although school presents a challenge to a person with a learning disability, research has shown that obtaining education can play a large role in the person's success rate. Improvement in skills commonly challenging to a person with a learning disability such as memory, perception, social functioning, and motivation can lead to successful employment. Knowledge by the employer of the disability and appropriate accommodations to be made can make the job more attainable.

CDMS Practice Test

1. What is the most common method for identifying malingering?

a. clinical interview
b. standardized psychological testing
c. clinical records
d. third-party interviews

2. In health insurance, what is the name for an amendment that increases or decreases benefits?

a. deductible
b. rider
c. copayment
d. premium

3. If an employee is found to have a disability he or she demonstrably had in an earlier job, which type of apportionment will be used with regard to workers compensation?

a. apportionment to historical factors
b. apportionment to off-the-job stressors
c. apportionment to the natural course of the disorder
d. apportionment to preexisting disability

4. Which of the following procedures is NOT a good way to mitigate injury?

a. maintaining a ready supply of antidotes to high-risk medications
b. simulation training
c. programming equipment to shut off in the event of a crisis
d. requiring employees to practice crisis response

5. The _____ of data is the degree to which they have appropriate specificity.

a. granularity
b. relevancy
c. accuracy
d. accessibility

6. Which financial statement indicates the assets, liabilities, and equity of a business?

a. statement of cash flows
b. balance sheet
c. income statement
d. statement of retained earnings

7. Diminished productivity at work, a common result of depression, is also known as

a. absenteeism.
b. dysthymia.
c. presenteeism.
d. malingering.

8. Which form of management makes the most use of statistical analysis?

a. risk management
b. utilization management
c. participatory management
d. quality assessment

9. Which of the following is NOT one of the specific categories of function outlined by the Social Security Administration?

a. activities of daily living
b. hand-eye coordination
c. social functioning
d. concentration, persistence, and pace

10. Which pay period is most often recommended by states?

a. monthly
b. twice monthly
c. weekly
d. twice weekly

11. Name one acknowledged weakness of the Global Assessment of Functioning (GAF) scale used by the DSM.

a. The GAF scale does not provide a valid measure of adaptive functioning.
b. The reliability of the GAF scale is correlated with the experience and knowledge of the rater.
c. The GAF scale does not assess mental impairment
d. The GAF scale does not produce an objective score.

12. Which dosimeter offers the most immediate measure of radiation exposure?

a. thermoluminescence detector
b. film badge
c. scintillation counter
d. pocket dosimeter

13. A simple but effective way for managers to obtain the support of team members is to

a. threaten punishment.
b. ask for it.
c. mandate it.
d. ignore the team members.

14. What type of workers compensation insurance are businesses required by state governments to purchase?

a. state-funded insurance
b. self-insurance
c. private insurance
d. all of these types of insurance are required by various states.

15. Which of the following is NOT one of the reasons why highly educated people tend to work to a more advanced age?

a. They have more debt.
b. They have less physically demanding jobs.
c. Their income increases at a greater rate as they acquire more experience.
d. They are healthier.

16. In which of the following situations would the Americans with Disabilities Act permit a business to deny employment to a disabled person?

a. moderate risk with minor consequences
b. very low risk with severe consequences
c. significant risk with minor consequences
d. minor risk with moderate consequences

17. Which of the following lower respiratory tract irritants is immediately dangerous to life and health at the lowest exposure level?

a. Cl_2
b. $COCl_2$
c. NO_2
d. O_3

18. Which of the following materials used in protective clothing provides the least protection against abrasion?

a. nitrile rubber
b. polyvinyl chloride
c. cotton
d. latex

19. An employee's high level stress leads to a myocardial infarction. What type of injury claim would this employee make?

a. physical-mental injury claim
b. mental-physical injury claim
c. mental-mental injury claim
d. physical-physical injury claim

20. During a meeting, the facilitator notices that one of the participants is getting agitated. After the meeting, what would be the best question for the facilitator to ask the participant?

a. "Why are you so angry?"
b. "What didn't you like about the meeting?"
c. "Were you feeling irritated during the meeting?"
d. "Don't you hate it when your coworkers act that way?"

21. Which of the following accommodations may be considered reasonable under the Americans with Disabilities Act?

a. providing treatment for an employee's condition
b. eliminating performance evaluations
c. providing a stress-free work environment
d. allowing an employee to work from home

22. Which filing system would be most appropriate for a workplace with a high risk of fire?

a. compressible filing system
b. open-shelf file system
c. filing cabinet
d. motorized revolving file system

23. Which of these disorders would be covered by the Americans with Disabilities Act?

a. kleptomania
b. dyslexia
c. pyromania
d. compulsive gambling

24. Which of the following factors is NOT included in a calculation of risk priority number?

a. severity of possible adverse effects
b. effectiveness of controls
c. likelihood of an adverse effect
d. cost of controls

25. What is the term for the percentage of people who have a disease at a particular time?

a. incidence rate
b. prevalence rate
c. morbidity rate
d. mortality rate

26. Which of the following is a standard characteristic of workers compensation legislation?

a. Benefits do not include hospital, medical, and rehabilitation expenses.
b. Negligence and fault are material to the validity of a claim.
c. Employees who are covered by workers compensation do not give up the right to sue the employer for damages.
d. The rules of procedure and evidence are relaxed in application.

27. Employee incentive programs should emphasize

a. adherence to established protocols.
b. excellent results.
c. improved cost savings.
d. reduction in adverse events.

28. Which aspect of financial health is indicated by the current ratio?

a. liquidity
b. solvency
c. profitability
d. indebtedness

29. Which of the following might result in a disability claim being allowed by the Social Security Administration?

a. The claimant's impairment does not prevent him from doing past relevant work.
b. The claimant is not currently engaged in substantial gainful activity.
c. The claimant's impairment does not prevent him from doing any other work.
d. The claimant does not have a severe impairment.

30. Which of the following conditions obliges an employer to discuss accommodations?

a. The employer knows that the employee has a disability.
b. The employer knows that the employee's disability is causing problems at work.
c. The employer knows that employee's disability prevents him or her from asking for accommodation.
d. All of the above conditions must be met.

31. Which of the following is NOT an advantage of local exhaust ventilation?

a. Hazards can be removed by shifting relatively small quantities of air.
b. It is rare that a large population will be exposed to a locally generated hazard.
c. Less energy is required to remove hazards.
d. The workstation does not need to be outfitted with a hood.

32. How long must a condition persist to be considered permanent, according to the American Medical Association?

a. 6 months
b. 12 months
c. 18 months
d. 24 months

33. Which of the following actions is NOT required of an employer who knows that an employee is physically disabled and desires an accommodation?

a. The employer must identify the key functions of the employee's job.
b. The employer must determine the accommodation that best serves the needs of the employer and employee.
c. The employer must transfer the employee to a more suitable position.
d. The employer should determine the precise physical or mental limitations of the employee.

34. Which piece of legislation created a program for detecting fraudulent health plans?

a. Health Insurance Portability and Accountability Act of 1996
b. Nursing Home Reform Act of 1987
c. Patient Self-Determination Act of 1990
d. Consolidated Omnibus Budget Reconciliation Act of 1995

35. The employees of a factory are exposed to noise of 95 dB for three hours, 90 dB for two hours, and 100 dB for one hour. The rest of the noise exposure is less than regulated levels. What calculation will be used to determine whether the factory is in compliance with OSHA noise regulations?

a. 95/3 + 90/2 + 100
b. 3/95 + 2/95 + 1/100
c. 4/3 + 8/2 + 2
d. 3/4 + 2/8 +1/2

36. An employee complains to an evaluator that his supervisor is singling him out for criticism. The evaluator believes that this complaint is the result of the employee's persecution bias, even though other employees have made similar comments about the supervisor. Which form of bias is the evaluator demonstrating?

a. advocacy bias
b. intrapsychic bias
c. extrapsychic bias
d. diagnosis bias

37. Which of the following is defined by the American Medical Association as a "significant deviation, loss, or loss of use of any body structure or body function in an individual with a health condition, disorder, or disease"?

a. handicap.
b. disability
c. injury
d. impairment

38. Which of the following is a healthy level of oxygen in the atmosphere?

a. 10%
b. 20%
c. 30%
d. 40%

39. Which of the following would be considered a legal rather than factual disability?

a. apnea
b. dyspraxia
c. mononucleosis
d. incarceration

40. How long must an employee's W-4 forms remain on file after the employee has been terminated?

a. six months
b. one year
c. two years
d. four years

41. What is the most important dimension of job burnout?

a. depersonalization
b. emotional exhaustion
c. feelings of inefficacy
d. cynicism

42. Which of the following upper respiratory tract irritants is immediately dangerous to life and health at the lowest dosage?

a. SO_2
b. HCl
c. NH_3
d. HF

43. Which of the following are NOT a component of the Health Belief model?

a. perceived susceptibilities
b. perceived risks
c. perceived barriers
d. perceived benefits

44. The part of the body most often affected in job-related disease is the

a. feet.
b. liver.
c. brain.
d. skin.

45. Which of the following terms describes an event that permanently worsens an underlying condition?

a. flare-up
b. exacerbation
c. recurrence
d. aggravation

46. Which of the following temperature measurements is required to determine whether a work environment is likely to cause heat stress?

a. dry bulb temperature
b. globe temperature
c. natural wet bulb temperature
d. All of the above

47. Which category of injury claim is associated with the most cases of fraud?

a. physical-physical
b. mental-physical
c. physical-mental
d. mental-mental

48. Which condition is the most common basis for a discrimination complaint under the Americans with Disabilities Act?

a. cancer
b. diabetes
c. orthopedic problems or injuries
d. depression

49. Which of the following statements about filing an SSDI claim is false?

a. Claimants maintain all their privacy rights after a claim is filed.
b. The first step in the filing of an SSDI claim is application to the SSA district office.
c. The responsibility for providing medical evidence of disability lies with the claimant.
d. The initial determination of disability is made by the Disability Determination Services, a state agency.

50. Which government body is primarily responsible for standardizing health information?

a. National Committee on Vital and Health Statistics
b. American Health Information Management Association
c. National Center for Health Statistics
d. Health and Human Services Data Council

Answer Key and Explanations

1. A: The most common method for identifying malingering is a clinical interview by an informed practitioner. There are specific interview structures that encourage presentation of verbal and behavioral characteristics of malingering. In order to make a final judgment, however, the evaluator may need to integrate standard psychological testing, clinical records, third-party interviews, and other documentation. Malingering presents in different ways: as exaggerated symptoms, imagined claims of discrimination, or feigned disability.

2. B: In health insurance, a rider is an amendment that increases or decreases benefits. A deductible is the minimum amount that the beneficiary of an insurance policy must incur before the insurance provider will pay for the remaining treatment. A copayment is a system in which the subscriber pays a certain amount out of his or her own pocket for every encounter with the healthcare system, with the remaining payment provided by the insurance company. A premium, finally, is a fixed payment made regularly to maintain insurance coverage.

3. D: If an employee is found to have a disability he or she demonstrably had in an earlier job, apportionment to pre-existing disability will be used to calculate workers compensation. This means that the entire disability will be apportioned to the pre-existing history. There is no such thing as apportionment to historical factors. Apportionment to off-the-job stressors is used when part of the workers disability can be assigned to personal, non-work-related issues. In these cases, a percentage of the disability is estimated for and apportioned to the off-the-job stressors. Apportionment to the natural course of the disorder is used for conditions that follow a typical and predictable course of deterioration. In these cases, a disability is apportioned according to the typical decline of function.

4. C: Programming equipment to shut off in the event of a crisis is not a good way to mitigate injury. Equipment should be programmed to default to the least-harmful setting, but in many cases shutting off is as harmful as operating incorrectly. For instance, a respirator should never default to an off position. All of the other answer choices represent excellent strategies to mitigate injury.

5. A: The granularity of data is the degree to which it has appropriate specificity. The relevancy of data is the extent to which it applies to the process or function for which it was collected. The accuracy of data is its correctness. The accessibility of data is the ease and legality with which it may be collected.

6. B: The balance sheet indicates the assets, liabilities, and equity of a business. The balance sheet, statement of cash flows, income statement, and statement of retained earnings are the four main financial reports produced by businesses. The statement of cash flows identifies how much cash is being earned and spent by operating, investing, and financing activities, respectively. The income statement compares the revenues and expenses of the business. The statement of retained earnings indicates how much of the company's profits were passed on the shareholders or reinvested in the business.

7. C: Diminished productivity at work is also known as presenteeism. Depression is a particularly common cause of presenteeism, in part because it is difficult to diagnose. Numerous studies have indicated the severe decline in productivity for depressed workers, though the total number of days missed from work may be quite typical. Absenteeism is persistent failure to show up at work. Dysthymia is low-grade depression. Malingering is the intentional exaggeration or invention of a disability for the purposes of avoiding work.

8. D: Quality assessment is the form of management that makes the most use of statistical analysis. The other two common forms of management are utilization management and risk management. In risk management, the administrators are more likely to use occurrence screening, while in utilization management they are more likely to use case management techniques. The purpose of quality assessment is to improve care and services by analyzing past performance. Utilization management focuses on effectively and efficiently using resources. Risk management is focused on avoiding liability.

9. B: Hand-eye coordination is not one of the specific categories of function outlined by the Social Security Administration. The SSA created this outline in order to systematize the diagnosis of impairment and disability. According to the model, there are four specific categories of function: activities of daily living; social functioning; concentration, persistence, and pace; and deterioration or decompensation in complex or work-like settings. Any person who has significant problems in one of these four categories may be considered to have a disability.

10. B: States most often recommend a twice monthly pay period. Many states actually require organizations of a certain size to use a twice monthly pay period, while others simply recommend doing so. Employers are required to withhold income tax for the selected pay period even when the employee does not work the entire time.

11. B: One acknowledged weakness of the Global Assessment of Functioning scale used by the Diagnostic and Statistical Manual of Mental Disorders is that its reliability is correlated with the experience and knowledge of the rater. In general, however, the GAF scale has proven both valid and reliable. The scale rates social, psychological, and occupational functioning from 1 to 100. The GAF scale is considered to be a valid measure of adaptive functioning. It does assess mental impairment; indeed, one of the main criticisms of the GFA scale is a perceived over-emphasis on mental impairment.

12. D: The pocket dosimeter offers the most immediate measure of radiation exposure. This device measures exposure to x-rays and gamma rays. It looks a bit like a pen, and can be read in real time. A thermoluminescence detector features a chip of lithium fluoride, which is stimulated by radiation. A film badge functions just like photographic film, except the film is developed by radiation instead of visible light. A scintillation counter is not a dosimeter. It indicates the level of radioactive emissions by measuring the amount of light created by the collision of radioactive emissions with certain liquids or crystals.

13. B: A simple but effective way for managers to obtain the support of team members is to ask for it. Unfortunately, many assertive managers feel that openly requesting buy-in from team members is a sign of weakness. On the contrary, the members of a team will be more likely to respond positively to a leader who is humble and capable of admitting that he or she needs help. Threats and coercion only antagonize subordinates. In large and successful businesses, team leaders are likely to be dealing with healthy egos. The best way to elicit the support of confident and independent employees is to request it straightforwardly.

14. D: Businesses are required by state governments to purchase state-funded insurance, self-insurance, or private insurance, depending on the state. In every state, however, businesses are required to purchase some form of workers compensation insurance.

15. A: The debt status of highly educated people is not one of the reasons why they tend to work to a more advanced age. However, highly educated workers do tend to earn more money as they gain experience. They also tend to be healthier and have less physically demanding jobs. The increasing number of highly educated workers will create ever more situations in which disability management is essential.

16. B: The Americans with Disabilities Act would permit a business to deny employment to a disabled person who posed a very low risk, but with severe consequences. The general rule for employing potentially dangerous people is that employers may decline to hire a person who poses a significant risk with a high probability of substantial harm. The courts have subsequently demonstrated that, in the calculation of risk, a balancing test may be used. In other words, a person may be denied employment if the risk is small, but the consequences of the risk would be severe. Likewise, a person may be denied employment if he or she imposes a severe risk, but with only minor or attendant consequences.

17. B: Of the given lower respiratory tract irritants, $COCl_2$ would be immediately dangerous to life and health at the lowest exposure level. Indeed, this chemical (also known as phosgene) can be deadly at a level as low as 2 parts per million. Cl_2 is immediately dangerous to life and health at levels of 25 parts per million. NO_2 is immediately dangerous at a level of 50 parts per million. O_3, otherwise known as ozone, is immediately dangerous at a level of 10 parts per million.

18. C: Of the given materials used in protective clothing, cotton provides the least protection against abrasion. Cotton protects well against many solids, but it should not be used for solvent protection. Nitrile rubber, on the other hand, provides good cut and abrasion resistance and protects well against nonpolar solvents, though it is ineffective against some polar solvents. Polyvinyl chloride provides good abrasion resistance and protects well against water solutions, acids, caustics, and some polar solvents. Latex, also known as natural rubber, protects well against polar solvents and water solutions, but is ineffective against nonpolar solvents. In general, latex provides good cut and abrasion resistance.

19. B: This employee would make a mental-physical injury claim. Many states have established three categories for psychiatric claims in workers compensation: physical-mental; mental-physical, and mental-mental. The order of the terms in these categories denotes the chronological relationship of the conditions. So, an employee whose high level of stress caused a myocardial infarction (heart attack) would file a mental-physical injury claim. All states permit physical-mental claims, but it is more difficult to register a mental-physical or mental-mental claim. There is no category for physical-physical injury claims.

20. C: In the given situation, the best question for the facilitator to ask would be, "Were you feeling irritated during the meeting?" This phrasing is appropriate because it does not make assumptions about the participant's feelings. It may be that the participant was not irritated, or was irritated by something unrelated to the meeting. In any case, the facilitator should not make any suppositions without first talking to the participant.

21. D: Under the Americans with Disabilities Act, it would be considered reasonable for an employer to accommodate an employee by allowing him or her to work from home, so long as this does not compromise the employee's performance and ability to meet the requirements of his or her job. The Americans with Disabilities Act does not consider it reasonable for an employer to be required to provide treatment for the employee's condition, to eliminate performance evaluations, or to provide a work environment that is completely free of stress. Moreover, employers will never be required by the ADA to create a new position, eliminate essential job functions, reduce performance standards, waive a uniformly applied disciplinary policy, provide indefinite or irregular leave, or arrange a transfer when no positions are available.

22. C: A filing cabinet system would be most appropriate for a workplace with a high risk of fire. Filing cabinets are widely available in fireproof versions, and generally are able to protect important records from environmental degradation. However, these cabinets can take up a great deal of space, and typically can only be opened one drawer at a time. A compressible filing system, on the other hand, is a manual or motorized system of parallel open-shelf files that move back and forth to create an opening. Compressible filing systems save a great deal of space, but are generate high maintenance costs. An open-shelf filing system is similar to a set of bookshelves: there is easy access to every file within the system, but all the records are open to environmental damage. A motorized revolving file system, finally, resembles a Ferris wheel. These systems are very space-efficient, but they are also precarious and must be kept organized in order to function properly.

23. B: Dyslexia is normally covered by the Americans with Disabilities Act. However, this and other learning disabilities may require extensive clinical interviews and neuropsychological testing to support a claim. It is necessary to demonstrate that the claimant is substantially impaired relative to the general population. The other answer choices are DSM disorders that are excluded from ADA coverage.

24. D: The cost of controls is not included in a calculation of risk priority number. A risk priority number, or RPN, is an objective picture of the importance of a particular danger to performance. It is calculated by rating on a scale from 1 to 10 the severity of each possible adverse effect (10 is the most severe), the likelihood of each of these effects (10 is the most certain to occur), and the effectiveness of possible controls (1 is the most effective), and then multiplying these three numbers.

25. B: Prevalence rate is the percentage of people who have a disease at a particular time. The incidence rate is calculated as the number of new cases of a disease during a specific interval divided by the total population during that interval. The morbidity rate is essentially the rate of complications for patients, though it should be noted that this rate also includes the prevalence and incidence of disease, as well as the comorbidity rate. The mortality rate could be any of a set of death rates, including the infant death rate, net death rate, or gross death rate.

26. D: In the standard workers compensation legislation, the rules of procedure and evidence are relaxed in application. The other answer choices are not characteristic of workers compensation legislation. The benefits afforded by this coverage typically include hospital, medical, and rehabilitation expenses, as well as between one-half and one-third of the average weekly wage. Negligence and fault are usually immaterial to the validity of the claim, as well as the assessment of its amount. Employees who are covered by workers comp give up the right to sue their employer for damages. Workers compensation is considered an exclusive remedy for this reason.

27. A: Employee incentive programs should emphasize adherence to established protocols. If performance protocols are clear and appropriate, they will define effective employee behavior. So long as employees abide by these protocols, their performance should be excellent. One characteristic of Six Sigma and other similar management philosophies is the emphasis on processes rather than result. If the processes are performed well, the results should take care of themselves. If incentives are tied to results, employees may be tempted to cheat or fudge their numbers. In some cases, perfect performance of the task may still result in error. Employees should not be penalized for such events. Instead, this sort of adverse situation should be cause for a reappraisal of the protocols.

28. A: The current ratio indicates liquidity, or the degree to which an organization's assets are in cash or can easily be converted to cash. It is calculated by dividing the current assets by the current liabilities. Current assets usually consist of cash, accounts receivable, and notes receivable. Current liabilities consist of accounts payable and notes payable.

29. B: If the claimant is not currently engaged in substantial gainful activity, his or her claim could still be allowed by the Social Security Administration. However, if the claimant's impairment does not prevent him or her from doing past relevant work (that is, tasks which have been an essential part of the job description in the past), the claim will be denied. Similarly, if the claimant's impairment does not prevent him or her from doing other work, or if the claimant does not have an impairment defined as severe by the Social Security Administration, then his or her claim will be denied.

30. D: An employer is obliged to discuss accommodations when he or she knows that the employee has a disability; knows or should know that the employee's disability is causing him or her problems at work; and knows or should know that the employee's disability prevents him or her from requesting an accommodation. The Americans with Disabilities Act states that when these conditions are met, the employer is required to meet with the employee as soon as possible.

31. D: Local exhaust ventilation systems do require that a hood be installed above the workstation. These hoods are used to intake the surrounding air and thereby remove the hazard. The other answer choices are advantages of a local exhaust ventilation system. These systems remove air at the point of hazard, so they are able to accomplish their mission by shifting relatively small quantities of air, and therefore using considerably less energy. Also, because they work in a confined area, they reduce the risk of exposing a large population to a locally generated hazard.

32. B: A condition must persist for 12 months to be considered permanent, according to the American Medical Association. More specifically, a condition is considered to be permanent if it persists even after the claimant has reached his or her maximum medical improvement (MMI). A claimant with such a condition may be eligible for palliative care, though it will be assumed that this care cannot greatly affect the underlying condition. A permanent condition exists when all reasonable medical treatment has been administered, and therefore further substantial improvement is unlikely.

33. C: An employer who knows that an employee is physically disabled and desires an accommodation is not required to transfer the employee to a more suitable position. However, the other three answer choices describe actions required by the Americans with Disabilities Act. Employers are required to identify the essential functions of the job; cooperate with the employee on a summary of physical or mental limitations; identify and assess potential accommodations; and select the accommodation that best serves the need of the employer and the employee. These actions should occur as soon as possible after a disability is identified.

34. A: The Health Insurance Portability and Accountability Act created a program for detecting fraudulent health plans. This act, passed in 1996 and implemented in

1998, generally improved the quality, access, and affordability of health insurance. The Nursing Home Reform Act, passed in 1987 and made effective in 1990, established minimum staffing requirements for long-term care facilities. The Patient Self-Determination Act, passed in 1990, mandated a wider dissemination of information to patients about their health options and rights. The Consolidated Omnibus Budget Reconciliation Act of 1985, commonly known as COBRA, established standards for the transfer and discharge of Medicaid and Medicare recipients.

35. D: The calculation that must be used here is 3/4 + 2/8 + 1/2 = 1 1/2. Because this value is greater than one, the factory is not in compliance with OSHA noise regulations. Compliance is determined by adding up a series of fractions, in which the numerator is the time exposed at a given level and the denominator is the permissible time of exposure at that level. Workers may only be exposed to sound at 95 dB for four hours per day, to sound at 90 dB for 8 hours per day, and to sound at 100 dB for 2 hours a day.

36. B: The evaluator is demonstrating intrapsychic bias. An intrapsychic bias exists when the evaluator overemphasizes the psychological (that is, internal) aspects of a case. This bias is particularly prevalent among psychoanalysts, psychiatrists, and psychologists. An advocacy bias exists when the evaluator has a vested interest in a particular diagnosis or treatment protocol. An extrapsychic bias exists when the evaluator places too much emphasis on external or environmental factors. Diagnosis bias exists when an evaluator feels compelled to offer some explanation for the employee's symptoms. Sometimes, an evaluator will believe that failing to make some positive assertion about the employee will indicate a lack of professional competence.

37. D: Impairment is defined by the American Medical Association as a "significant deviation, loss, or loss of use of an Impairment is defined by the American Medical Association as a "significant deviation, loss, or loss of use of an body structure or body function in an individual with a health condition, disorder, or disease." An impairment can be measured and is related to a medical condition. Disability, on the other hand, is defined by the American Medical Association as any "activity limitations and/or participation restrictions in an individual with a health condition, disorder, or disease." A mild impairment could lead to a significant, even permanent disability. By contrast, a severe impairment could fail to cause a significant disability.

38. B: 20% is a healthy level of oxygen in the atmosphere. People will have difficulty breathing when the oxygen level sinks to 14%. Consciousness is lost at 10%, and death is likely when the oxygen level falls to 8%. According to OSHA, workplaces must have at least a 19.5% oxygen level, or else workers require a special breathing apparatus. On the other hand, excessively high oxygen levels can create a risk of fire or explosion. Oxygen levels of 23% or more are considered excessive, and, indeed, OSHA caps acceptable oxygen levels at 23.5%.

39. D: Incarceration would be considered a legal rather than factual disability. Legal disability is an inability or incapacity to perform job duties because of legal issues, as for instance license suspension or incarceration. Factual disabilities, on the other hand, are related to medical impairments caused by illness or injury.

40. D: An employee's W-4 forms must remain on file for four years after the employee has been terminated. A W-4 form is where an employee indicates his or her tax withholding status. Both federal and state laws require the retention of W-4 forms. There are also federal and state laws requiring companies to maintain W-2s and copies of filed tax forms.

41. B: The most important dimension of job burnout is emotional exhaustion. An employee will experience emotional exhaustion when an overwhelming workload consistently depletes his or her energy resources. The other answer choices are common but slightly less important dimensions of job burnout. A burned-out employee will often demonstrate depersonalization and cynicism, meaning that he or she will express negative opinions about the organization and will become personally detached from the success of the institution and from the quality of his or her work. Finally, a burned-out employee will often be beset by feelings of inefficacy, meaning that he or she will perceive a personal lack of influence or effectiveness.

42. D: Of the given upper respiratory tract irritants, HF is immediately dangerous to life and health at the lowest dosage. At a level of only 20 ppm, HF can cause permanent damage to the human organism. The permissible exposure level for this compound is 3 parts per million (ppm). The permissible exposure level is a time-weighted average that assumes an eight-hour day. SO_2, HCl, and NH_3 are immediately dangerous to life or health at levels of 100 ppm.

43. B: Perceived risks are not a component of the Health Belief model. This model of health behavior has three components: perceived susceptibilities, perceived barriers, and perceived benefits. In other words, a person's health behavior is influenced by how vulnerable he or she believes him or herself to be, how difficult he or she believes taking positive action would be, and the potential rewards of taking these positive actions.

44. D: The part of the body most often affected in job-related disease is the skin. Indeed, some estimates suggest that two-thirds of all health issues reported on the job are associated with the skin. The majority of claims paid by insurance companies are related to industrial dermatitis. Moreover, skin problems are often undercounted because loopholes in the OSHA requirements allow some minor injuries to be unreported if only first aid is required.

45. D: An aggravation is an event that permanently worsens an underlying condition. Exacerbations, flare-ups, and recurrences, on the other hand, are events that only temporarily worsen a condition. These are the definitions advanced by the American Medical Association.

46. D: Dry bulb temperature, globe temperature, and natural wet bulb temperature are all required to determine whether a work environment is likely to cause heat stress. These three measures are required to create the Wet Bulb Globe Temperature index. Dry bulb temperature is the measure obtained with an ordinary thermometer. Globe temperature is obtained by inserting the thermometer bulb into a small copper sphere painted black on the outside. Typically, globe temperature will be higher than dry bulb temperature. Natural wet bulb temperature is obtained by using a thermometer with a wick that transports water to the thermometer bulb. Typically, the evaporation of this water will cool the bulb, so the wet bulb temperature is usually lower than the dry bulb temperature.

47. D: Mental-mental injury claims are associated with the most cases of fraud. It is easy to see why this is: mental disabilities are more difficult to observe and measure objectively, and therefore are more susceptible to malingering and misrepresentation. Unfortunately, one of the consequences of the elevated risk of fraud in mental-mental injury claims is greater skepticism about mental illness. For employees with legitimate mental problems, this creates an unhealthy atmosphere of suspicion and shame.

48. C: Orthopedic problems or injuries are the most common basis for a discrimination complaint under the Americans with Disabilities Act. Indeed, in 2007 almost 16% of all ADA discrimination claims were related to orthopedic problems or injuries. The second most common basis for a discrimination complaint is depression, followed by hearing and vision impairments, diabetes, bipolar disorder, and cancer. These findings indicate that there is still a persistent bias against employees with mental disabilities.

49. A: Claimants do not maintain all of their privacy rights after a claim is filed. Indeed, the filing of a claim is tantamount to the waiver of privilege or privacy claims that would otherwise apply to medical and other records. Claimants are required to provide any necessary medical evidence for their condition. The other answer choices are true statements. The first step in the filing of an SSDI claim is the submission of an application to the SSA district office. This claim will then be referred to Disability Determination Services, a state agency that makes the initial determination of disability. The claimant is responsible for providing medical evidence of his or her condition.

50. A: The National Committee on Vital and Health Statistics (NCVHS) is primarily responsible for standardizing health information. The NCVHS is a component of the Department of Health and Human Services. It encourages public and private entities to collaborate on a uniform and efficient health information system. The American Health Information Management Association (AHIMA) is a professional development organization that offers training, certification, and research opportunities to those who are interested. The National Center for Health Statistics (NCHS) is a division of the Centers for Disease Control and Prevention (CDC). The NCHS is an aggregator and disseminator of vital and health statistics. The Health and

Human Services Data Council organizes the data collection efforts in both medical and nonmedical areas.

How to Overcome Test Anxiety

Just the thought of taking a test is enough to make most people a little nervous. A test is an important event that can have a long-term impact on your future, so it's important to take it seriously and it's natural to feel anxious about performing well. But just because anxiety is normal, that doesn't mean that it's helpful in test taking, or that you should simply accept it as part of your life. Anxiety can have a variety of effects. These effects can be mild, like making you feel slightly nervous, or severe, like blocking your ability to focus or remember even a simple detail.

If you experience test anxiety—whether severe or mild—it's important to know how to beat it. To discover this, first you need to understand what causes test anxiety.

Causes of Test Anxiety

While we often think of anxiety as an uncontrollable emotional state, it can actually be caused by simple, practical things. One of the most common causes of test anxiety is that a person does not feel adequately prepared for their test. This feeling can be the result of many different issues such as poor study habits or lack of organization, but the most common culprit is time management. Starting to study too late, failing to organize your study time to cover all of the material, or being distracted while you study will mean that you're not well prepared for the test. This may lead to cramming the night before, which will cause you to be physically and mentally exhausted for the test. Poor time management also contributes to feelings of stress, fear, and hopelessness as you realize you are not well prepared but don't know what to do about it.

Other times, test anxiety is not related to your preparation for the test but comes from unresolved fear. This may be a past failure on a test, or poor performance on tests in general. It may come from comparing yourself to others who seem to be performing better or from the stress of living up to expectations. Anxiety may be driven by fears of the future—how failure on this test would affect your educational and career goals. These fears are often completely irrational, but they can still negatively impact your test performance.

Elements of Test Anxiety

As mentioned earlier, test anxiety is considered to be an emotional state, but it has physical and mental components as well. Sometimes you may not even realize that you are suffering from test anxiety until you notice the physical symptoms. These can include trembling hands, rapid heartbeat, sweating, nausea, and tense muscles. Extreme anxiety may lead to fainting or vomiting. Obviously, any of these symptoms can have a negative impact on testing. It is important to recognize them as soon as they begin to occur so that you can address the problem before it damages your performance.

The mental components of test anxiety include trouble focusing and inability to remember learned information. During a test, your mind is on high alert, which can help you recall information and stay focused for an extended period of time. However, anxiety interferes with your mind's natural processes, causing you to blank out, even on the questions you know well. The strain of testing during anxiety makes it difficult to stay focused, especially on a test that may take several hours. Extreme anxiety can take a huge mental toll, making it difficult not only to recall test information but even to understand the test questions or pull your thoughts together.

Effects of Test Anxiety

Test anxiety is like a disease—if left untreated, it will get progressively worse. Anxiety leads to poor performance, and this reinforces the feelings of fear and failure, which in turn lead to poor performances on subsequent tests. It can grow from a mild nervousness to a crippling condition. If allowed to progress, test anxiety can have a big impact on your schooling, and consequently on your future.

Test anxiety can spread to other parts of your life. Anxiety on tests can become anxiety in any stressful situation, and blanking on a test can turn into panicking in a job situation. But fortunately, you don't have to let anxiety rule your testing and determine your grades. There are a number of relatively simple steps you can take to move past anxiety and function normally on a test and in the rest of life.

Physical Steps for Beating Test Anxiety

While test anxiety is a serious problem, the good news is that it can be overcome. It doesn't have to control your ability to think and remember information. While it may take time, you can begin taking steps today to beat anxiety.

Just as your first hint that you may be struggling with anxiety comes from the physical symptoms, the first step to treating it is also physical. Rest is crucial for having a clear, strong mind. If you are tired, it is much easier to give in to anxiety. But if you establish good sleep habits, your body and mind will be ready to perform optimally, without the strain of exhaustion. Additionally, sleeping well helps you to retain information better, so you're more likely to recall the answers when you see the test questions.

Getting good sleep means more than going to bed on time. It's important to allow your brain time to relax. Take study breaks from time to time so it doesn't get overworked, and don't study right before bed. Take time to rest your mind before trying to rest your body, or you may find it difficult to fall asleep.

Along with sleep, other aspects of physical health are important in preparing for a test. Good nutrition is vital for good brain function. Sugary foods and drinks may give a burst of energy but this burst is followed by a crash, both physically and emotionally. Instead, fuel your body with protein and vitamin-rich foods.

Also, drink plenty of water. Dehydration can lead to headaches and exhaustion, especially if your brain is already under stress from the rigors of the test. Particularly if your test is a long one, drink water during the breaks. And if possible, take an energy-boosting snack to eat between sections.

Along with sleep and diet, a third important part of physical health is exercise. Maintaining a steady workout schedule is helpful, but even taking 5-minute study breaks to walk can help get your blood pumping faster and clear your head. Exercise also releases endorphins, which contribute to a positive feeling and can help combat test anxiety.

When you nurture your physical health, you are also contributing to your mental health. If your body is healthy, your mind is much more likely to be healthy as well. So take time to rest, nourish your body with healthy food and water, and get moving as much as possible. Taking these physical steps will make you stronger and more able to take the mental steps necessary to overcome test anxiety.

Mental Steps for Beating Test Anxiety

Working on the mental side of test anxiety can be more challenging, but as with the physical side, there are clear steps you can take to overcome it. As mentioned earlier, test anxiety often stems from lack of preparation, so the obvious solution is to prepare for the test. Effective studying may be the most important weapon you have for beating test anxiety, but you can and should employ several other mental tools to combat fear.

First, boost your confidence by reminding yourself of past success—tests or projects that you aced. If you're putting as much effort into preparing for this test as you did for those, there's no reason you should expect to fail here. Work hard to prepare; then trust your preparation.

Second, surround yourself with encouraging people. It can be helpful to find a study group, but be sure that the people you're around will encourage a positive attitude. If you spend time with others who are anxious or cynical, this will only contribute to your own anxiety. Look for others who are motivated to study hard from a desire to succeed, not from a fear of failure.

Third, reward yourself. A test is physically and mentally tiring, even without anxiety, and it can be helpful to have something to look forward to. Plan an activity following the test, regardless of the outcome, such as going to a movie or getting ice cream.

When you are taking the test, if you find yourself beginning to feel anxious, remind yourself that you know the material. Visualize successfully completing the test. Then take a few deep, relaxing breaths and return to it. Work through the questions carefully but with confidence, knowing that you are capable of succeeding.

Developing a healthy mental approach to test taking will also aid in other areas of life. Test anxiety affects more than just the actual test—it can be damaging to your mental health and even contribute to depression. It's important to beat test anxiety before it becomes a problem for more than testing.

Study Strategy

Being prepared for the test is necessary to combat anxiety, but what does being prepared look like? You may study for hours on end and still not feel prepared. What you need is a strategy for test prep. The next few pages outline our recommended steps to help you plan out and conquer the challenge of preparation.

Step 1: Scope Out the Test

Learn everything you can about the format (multiple choice, essay, etc.) and what will be on the test. Gather any study materials, course outlines, or sample exams that may be available. Not only will this help you to prepare, but knowing what to expect can help to alleviate test anxiety.

Step 2: Map Out the Material

Look through the textbook or study guide and make note of how many chapters or sections it has. Then divide these over the time you have. For example, if a book has 15 chapters and you have five days to study, you need to cover three chapters each day. Even better, if you have the time, leave an extra day at the end for overall review after you have gone through the material in depth.

If time is limited, you may need to prioritize the material. Look through it and make note of which sections you think you already have a good grasp on, and which need review. While you are studying, skim quickly through the familiar sections and take more time on the challenging parts. Write out your plan so you don't get lost as you go. Having a written plan also helps you feel more in control of the study, so anxiety is less likely to arise from feeling overwhelmed at the amount to cover.

Step 3: Gather Your Tools

Decide what study method works best for you. Do you prefer to highlight in the book as you study and then go back over the highlighted portions? Or do you type out notes of the important information? Or is it helpful to make flashcards that you can carry with you? Assemble the pens, index cards, highlighters, post-it notes, and any other materials you may need so you won't be distracted by getting up to find things while you study.

If you're having a hard time retaining the information or organizing your notes, experiment with different methods. For example, try color-coding by subject with colored pens, highlighters, or post-it notes. If you learn better by hearing, try recording yourself reading your notes so you can listen while in the car, working out, or simply sitting at your desk. Ask a friend to quiz you from your flashcards, or try teaching someone the material to solidify it in your mind.

Step 4: Create Your Environment

It's important to avoid distractions while you study. This includes both the obvious distractions like visitors and the subtle distractions like an uncomfortable chair (or a too-comfortable couch that makes you want to fall asleep). Set up the best study environment possible: good lighting and a comfortable work area. If background music helps you focus, you may want to turn it on, but otherwise keep the room quiet. If you are using a computer to take notes, be sure you don't have any other windows open, especially applications like social media, games, or anything else that could distract you. Silence your phone and turn off notifications. Be sure to keep water close by so you stay hydrated while you study (but avoid unhealthy drinks and snacks).

Also, take into account the best time of day to study. Are you freshest first thing in the morning? Try to set aside some time then to work through the material. Is your mind clearer in the afternoon or evening? Schedule your study session then. Another method is to study at the same time of day that you will take the test, so that your brain gets used to working on the material at that time and will be ready to focus at test time.

Step 5: Study!

Once you have done all the study preparation, it's time to settle into the actual studying. Sit down, take a few moments to settle your mind so you can focus, and begin to follow your study plan. Don't give in to distractions or let yourself procrastinate. This is your time to prepare so you'll be ready to fearlessly approach the test. Make the most of the time and stay focused.

Of course, you don't want to burn out. If you study too long you may find that you're not retaining the information very well. Take regular study breaks. For example, taking five minutes out of every hour to walk briskly, breathing deeply and swinging your arms, can help your mind stay fresh.

As you get to the end of each chapter or section, it's a good idea to do a quick review. Remind yourself of what you learned and work on any difficult parts. When you feel that you've mastered the material, move on to the next part. At the end of your study session, briefly skim through your notes again.

But while review is helpful, cramming last minute is NOT. If at all possible, work ahead so that you won't need to fit all your study into the last day. Cramming overloads your brain with more information than it can process and retain, and your tired mind may struggle to recall even previously learned information when it is overwhelmed with last-minute study. Also, the urgent nature of cramming and the stress placed on your brain contribute to anxiety. You'll be more likely to go to the test feeling unprepared and having trouble thinking clearly.

So don't cram, and don't stay up late before the test, even just to review your notes at a leisurely pace. Your brain needs rest more than it needs to go over the information again. In fact, plan to finish your studies by noon or early afternoon the day before the test. Give your brain the rest of the day to relax or focus on other things, and get a good night's sleep. Then you will be fresh for the test and better able to recall what you've studied.

Step 6: Take a Practice Test

Many courses offer sample tests, either online or in the study materials. This is an excellent resource to check whether you have mastered the material, as well as to prepare for the test format and environment.

Check the test format ahead of time: the number of questions, the type (multiple choice, free response, etc.), and the time limit. Then create a plan for working through them. For example, if you have 30 minutes to take a 60-question test, your limit is 30 seconds per question. Spend less time on the questions you know well so that you can take more time on the difficult ones.

If you have time to take several practice tests, take the first one open book, with no time limit. Work through the questions at your own pace and make sure you fully understand them. Gradually work up to taking a test under test conditions: sit at a desk with all study materials put away and set a timer. Pace yourself to make sure you finish the test with time to spare and go back to check your answers if you have time.

After each test, check your answers. On the questions you missed, be sure you understand why you missed them. Did you misread the question (tests can use tricky wording)? Did you forget the information? Or was it something you hadn't learned? Go back and study any shaky areas that the practice tests reveal.

Taking these tests not only helps with your grade, but also aids in combating test anxiety. If you're already used to the test conditions, you're less likely to worry about it, and working through tests until you're scoring well gives you a confidence boost. Go through the practice tests until you feel comfortable, and then you can go into the test knowing that you're ready for it.

Test Tips

On test day, you should be confident, knowing that you've prepared well and are ready to answer the questions. But aside from preparation, there are several test day strategies you can employ to maximize your performance.

First, as stated before, get a good night's sleep the night before the test (and for several nights before that, if possible). Go into the test with a fresh, alert mind rather than staying up late to study.

Try not to change too much about your normal routine on the day of the test. It's important to eat a nutritious breakfast, but if you normally don't eat breakfast at all, consider eating just a protein bar. If you're a coffee drinker, go ahead and have your normal coffee. Just make sure you time it so that the caffeine doesn't wear off right in the middle of your test. Avoid sugary beverages, and drink enough water to stay hydrated but not so much that you need a restroom break 10 minutes into the test. If your test isn't first thing in the morning, consider going for a walk or doing a light workout before the test to get your blood flowing.

Allow yourself enough time to get ready, and leave for the test with plenty of time to spare so you won't have the anxiety of scrambling to arrive in time. Another reason to be early is to select a good seat. It's helpful to sit away from doors and windows, which can be distracting. Find a good seat, get out your supplies, and settle your mind before the test begins.

When the test begins, start by going over the instructions carefully, even if you already know what to expect. Make sure you avoid any careless mistakes by following the directions.

Then begin working through the questions, pacing yourself as you've practiced. If you're not sure on an answer, don't spend too much time on it, and don't let it shake your confidence. Either skip it and come back later, or eliminate as many wrong answers as possible and guess among the remaining ones. Don't dwell on these questions as you continue—put them out of your mind and focus on what lies ahead.

Be sure to read all of the answer choices, even if you're sure the first one is the right answer. Sometimes you'll find a better one if you keep reading. But don't second-guess yourself if you do immediately know the answer. Your gut instinct is usually right. Don't let test anxiety rob you of the information you know.

If you have time at the end of the test (and if the test format allows), go back and review your answers. Be cautious about changing any, since your first instinct tends to be correct, but make sure you didn't misread any of the questions or accidentally mark the wrong answer choice. Look over any you skipped and make an educated guess.

At the end, leave the test feeling confident. You've done your best, so don't waste time worrying about your performance or wishing you could change anything. Instead, celebrate the successful completion of this test. And finally, use this test to learn how to deal with anxiety even better next time.

Review Video: Test Anxiety
Visit mometrix.com/academy and enter code: 100340

Important Qualification

Not all anxiety is created equal. If your test anxiety is causing major issues in your life beyond the classroom or testing center, or if you are experiencing troubling physical symptoms related to your anxiety, it may be a sign of a serious physiological or psychological condition. If this sounds like your situation, we strongly encourage you to seek professional help.

Online Resources

Due to our efforts to try to keep this book to a manageable length, we've created a link that will give you access to all of your online resources:

mometrix.com/resources719/cdms

It's Your Moment, Let's Celebrate It!

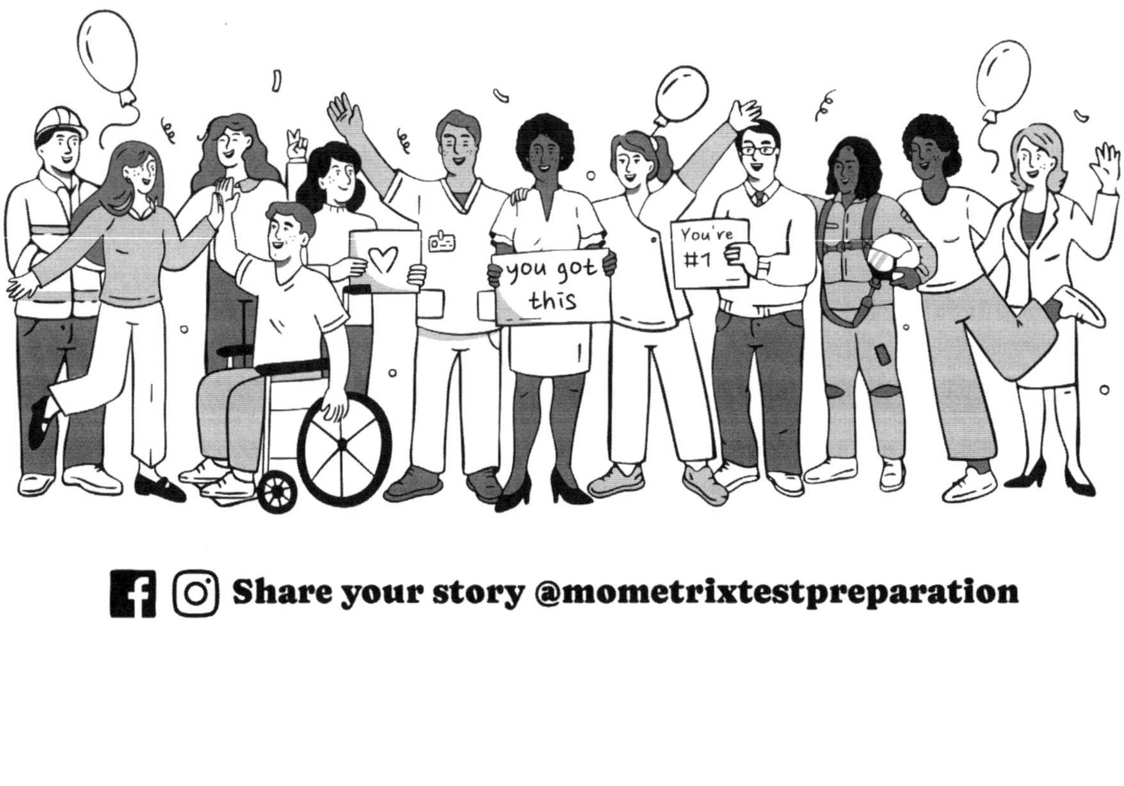

Share your story @mometrixtestpreparation